MY
NAME
IS
JHON

MY NAME IS JHON

AN ATYPICAL STORY OF SUCCESS

John Brennan

Gill Books

Gill Books
Hume Avenue
Park West
Dublin 12
www.gillbooks.ie

Gill Books is an imprint of M.H. Gill and Co.

978 07171 9140 6

Edited by Shane Dunphy
Copyedited by Susan McKeever
Proofread by Neil Burkey
Design and print origination by O'K Graphic Design, Dublin

Printed by CPI Group (UK) Ltd, Croydon, CR0 4YY.
This book is typeset in 11/17 pt Sabon.

A CIP catalogue record for this book is available from the British Library.

5 4 3 2 1

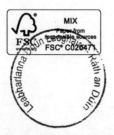

Thanks to my mother and father for understanding that underachievement at school is not the end of the world. Thanks also to my brothers and sisters, and to Gwen, Adam and Ruth. Finally, to all whose paths I have crossed, particularly in the businesses, thanks for the support – even if you didn't know you were and still are giving it.

CONTENTS

INTRODUCTION

I am not a reader and never had any desire to write a book, but in November of 2019 I found myself, at the age of 54, with time on my hands and nothing to do for the first time in my life. It was a strange feeling.

I decided to fill it with what some would call 'journaling'. Those quickly scribbled pages gradually transformed into the book you have before you, a book that was not written to be published or to make money, but simply to pass time.

The reason it made its way onto the shelves of bookshops is due to a fondly held wish that perhaps just one stressed parent, or maybe a single anxious teenager might recognise themselves and be inspired through reading its contents not to stress too much about life: it is simpler than most of us think, and can be great fun if we follow our instincts instead of doing what society thinks we should do. I have, through my work in the hospitality industry, met many wonderful young people who have been mislabelled by the educational system or forced, through peer pressure, into aspiring to be something they are not.

I would be very happy if my time in front of the computer went some way to changing that, even for just one person, as one person changed me.

Those who, like me, are not big readers needn't worry – this will be an easy read with no big words to worry about (words like library – but you'll understand the importance of that word later in the book, it's a funny little one). You will see as the story progresses, I'm not a fan of overly complicated language.

Which just leaves me to say: thank you for being here, and I hope you enjoy your stay.

Jhon

PROLOGUE

A Message from the Past

This is the story of my life, but I'm going to begin it with a death, and with something important I learned as a result.

My mother, Maura, passed away on 17 January 2020. She was 97 years old and lived a full and contented life. On the day before she died, she spent the morning having visits from neighbours, the afternoon chatting with family over the phone and had tea with friends that evening. Her death brought us great sadness, but if there is a good way to pass out of this world, she found it. Ninety-seven glorious years, living at home, never really sick in her life and fully mobile and mentally conscious until that week – most of us would settle happily for such a passing.

She and my father, Tom, who died in 1988, lived in a house they'd built on land attached to my mother's family farm. They moved to Sligo from Dublin when I was in my early teens. It's a move I will always be grateful for, as I wouldn't be the person I am if we'd stayed in Ireland's capital. The West of Ireland, its people and its personality, formed me and took me on a fantastic journey that still isn't finished, I hope.

I'm well aware a lot of my neighbours consider me a blow-in, but at the same time, if I were to pick up the phone and call any of them for help, they'd be over in five minutes to assist me with whatever I needed, no questions asked.

That's what people in this part of the world are like. And it's a quality I've come to treasure. Without it, the businesses I've built, on my own and with my older brother, Francis, wouldn't have been possible. Everything I've done has been based around that particular sense of warmth, ingenuity and stubbornness that makes West of Ireland people unique. And dare I say it, Kerry people in particular.

If you'd asked me ten years ago, I'd have told you that ingenuity and open-hearted friendliness were what inspired me to follow my dreams into the hotel trade. But my mother's death showed me that would have been wrong. And here's why.

After Mum passed, my nephew, Paul, moved into her house. He's planning to get married, and the family thought we would all sleep a bit easier knowing someone was on-site, looking after the property. The arrangement was a win-win for everyone. Paul insisted that, while he was in the house, he'd sort through the countless odds and ends my parents had collected over a lifetime together. He knew there would be all kinds of things different family members would want and others that could be either put in storage or just thrown out. I'm not particularly sentimental, but I was glad not to have to do that job, which was bound to be an emotional one. I'd called my parents' house 'home' for fifteen years, so there was no way I could do it without all kinds of memories flooding back, whether I wanted them to or not. So I whole-heartedly encouraged Paul to get stuck in to decluttering.

One evening, I got a call from my nephew saying he was sending me an email, as there was something he felt I should see.

'Have a look at it, and tell me what you think,' he said.

The email had my father's name on it, and the name of an architectural firm. I opened the attachment and found plans for the most magnificent hotel. I'm extremely interested in design and the art and creativity that goes into creating the spaces we all live in, and I knew as soon as I laid eyes on this that it was a work of great insight and beauty. I was reminded of some of the structures Frank Lloyd Wright had created, constructions I'd travelled to the United States just to see.

I emailed him back:

'What is this, Paul?'

Paul dispensed with emailing and just phoned instead. He told me these were plans my dad had come up with in 1964 for a hotel on my mother's family land in Sligo.

There wasn't a level bit of earth in the whole place, but it was in a gorgeous location overlooking Loch Gill, with views of Inisfree and Beezie's Island. Viewing the spot now with a lifetime of experience in the business behind me, I can see how it could have been a huge success.

I sat there gazing at the drawings, and I was completely blown away. By today's standards, the building is stunning and sensitively designed, but in the sixties, it would have seemed outrageously ambitious. In fact, it would have been unlike anything that existed in Ireland at that time.

And that was what really caused me to stop and think.

The biggest issue Francis and I face on our TV show, *At Your Service*, in which we help people out whose hospitality businesses have run into trouble, is that they are often fixated on what the business down the road is doing. If their neighbour is offering a successful carvery lunch, they want to do the same. If they're doing guided birdwatching tours of the nearby woodlands, then our struggling hoteliers think they should too. One of the first things I have to teach them is that the greatest selling point you can have is to be different – to bring something to the table no one else has.

Somehow, in 1964, in an Ireland crippled with unemployment and lack of education, a much smaller and more insular Ireland than the one of today, my father knew that simple truth. He strove to be completely different. He thought outside the box.

Ultimately, and a little sadly, he and my mum decided it was too great a gamble and Dad chose not to make his hotel dreams a reality. Which may also be a blessing. I was born in 1965, and if they ended up going ahead with the hotel it's quite likely they would have been much too preoccupied to even think about adding to their family.

Who'd have thought I'd be grateful for a hotel that never was? Or perhaps after reading this you might think, 'Pity they didn't build the hotel!'

That night, as I showed my children, Adam and Ruth, my father's 60-year-old designs, and saw them being moved by their grandfather's vision and inventiveness, I was struck by the legacy he had left me. I'd always seen him as a sound businessman – he ran a local shop in the community in Dublin where we lived – and as someone who passed on a sense of independence and an attention to detail, not to mention hard work. But I never knew until that moment that he had a dream of something bigger. And that he passed that dream on to me.

PART ONE

Early Years

Balally Drive

I was born in 1965 in Balally Drive, a small housing estate between Dundrum and Sandyford in South County Dublin.

I was the youngest of five children. The next oldest, Susan, is eight years my senior, which suggests I was something of an afterthought. I was probably doted on for the first few months, but there are no photos whatsoever of me until I was about six. Maybe I was an ugly baby – but then, maybe not. Let's just agree I improved with age.

Dad owned a grocery shop in Stepaside, a village on the southern outskirts of Dublin City. He worked very hard. Business was always a presence in our home, as yesterday's takings influenced every aspect of what we did today: what we ate, the myriad small jobs we needed to accomplish to support his efforts in the shop, and particularly what time my parents got to sit down for the evening.

Mum looked after us and we had a very happy house. She always said we could never be rich as we ate all the profits from the shop. We didn't have any money, but we did have a good life as we wanted for nothing. We didn't need sun holidays, weekends away in luxury hotels or cars, boats or motorbikes. All those things could come later.

Balally Drive was a small cul de sac of 47 semi-detached bungalows that had been built in the 1950s. At that time, the area was very much on the edge of Dublin, almost in the countryside, and it was surrounded by fields, narrow laneways and woods. In those days it was a community, where friendships grew and lifelong family ties were made.

I was by far the youngest in our area: most of the children on our road were 10 to 15 years older than me. So while there were occasional games of 'kerbs' played on the road (a game involving standing on opposite sides of the road and attempting to bounce a football back at yourself by hitting it at just the correct angle on the kerb of the footpath), I was normally the one looking on from the sitting room window.

I don't remember being lonely, but saying that, I never had a band of friends to play with, which seems odd and a little bit empty when I look back on it. At the time it never registered with me, as that was simply how my life was. And it gave me a reason to want to go to school. Which became very important as I got older, and learning became more of a challenge.

Educational Speedbumps

My primary education took me just up the road to a new school, built to facilitate both the extension of the estate and the expansion of Dublin. The fields, lanes and trees were slowly starting to disappear.

My poor mother did her best to set me up for each day of learning, cooking eggs three different ways and laying out cereals and juice before walking me up the road to where I was supposed to be absorbing wisdom. But I'd fly out the door having eaten nothing, so most days she would return to find her efforts lying in exactly the same position, untouched, still looking like the buffet we have all come to recognise from mornings in hotels. I'm not sure if it was fear of school or just general disinterest, but I was never a big breakfast fan.

As I was starting out on my educational journey, other changes were happening at home. At this stage Damien, the eldest, had left home to join the Marist Priests in Milltown. Damien, just like Francis and I, had attended Catholic University School (CUS) in Lesson Street, where he did very well. I think we all knew he felt a calling for the religious life, so it was no surprise when he told us he was entering the seminary. Milltown was where my father hailed from, so the Marist Monastery, which is still situated there, was an obvious choice.

Just as Damien was taking up Holy Orders, the garage was converted into a bedroom for Francis. He attended

Cathal Brugha Street to study Hotel Management, and it was decided he needed some independence and space, so he was given the garage as a kind of student bedsit – one still attached to the house, but it meant he had some peace while he was studying.

The girls, Catherine and Susan, went to boarding school in Arklow which, while not really terribly far to travel by today's standards, felt like another world away back then. They came home most weekends, but during the week I was basically home alone, albeit with a brother in the garage. With no friends on the street to play with, and school becoming increasingly challenging for me, my life became one of quiet solitude. Which sounds more miserable than it was, as I was actually quite busy.

Days revolved around school and homework. I was about seven years old when I became obsessed by motorbikes. I don't really know where this interest came from – I remember sitting at home, gazing out the sitting room window, and seeing one of the young men who lived nearby cruising past on a BSA he had gotten second-hand somewhere, and feeling a rush of real excitement. It was very different from all the other vehicles on our road – faster and sleeker and maybe just a little bit dangerous.

As the youngest member of a shopkeeper's family, the idea that I might one day be speeding around atop a machine like that seemed very far-fetched indeed, but it was something I dreamed about. As I gazed out the window at the older kids playing, I imagined myself whizzing past them all on a shiny, chrome-trimmed bike.

It got so that motorbikes were all I could either think of

or talk about. Our great family friends, the Redmonds in Ranelagh, took pity on me and Mary Redmond would give me bundles of old motorbike magazines her son Michael bought monthly, which I would pore over, absorbing each photograph they contained and memorising the names and model numbers of every bike I came across.

A lot of the hours I spent in school were taken up with thinking about bikes, as school was rapidly becoming a place where I dreamed classes away and counted down the clock to the break or, even better, to home time. I never hated going, because in school there were loads of other people my age to play with. Learning, however, never featured as a reason for attending, as nothing captured my imagination or connected with me. It was all book-based, and I had no interest whatsoever.

The truth behind my disinterest was that almost immediately, I found reading and writing a challenge. The words would swim and spin on the pages put in front of me. The teacher would slowly and patiently spell them for me, sounding out the letters, but she might as well have been speaking a foreign language. I could not grasp what was going on, and most teachers eventually just gave up on me. I'd be left down the back of the class to get on with my daydreaming, and this suited me (and probably the teacher) down to the ground.

My poor, beleaguered mother did all she could to motivate me, but I just didn't get what school was about. I couldn't see the point. I didn't care about the silly storybooks – who cared if Spot caught the ball or what Dick and Jane bought at the market? – and how did knowing when the Battle of Hastings took place help me in any way? It was all baloney.

I don't know how my mother coped with me. If I didn't start my homework the minute I came in from school it wouldn't get done. If even half an hour was allowed to pass, you could forget it, all overtures of an educational nature would fall on deaf ears. So I drifted, much to my mother's and father's heartache, I am sure.

MOTORBIKES

Motorbikes, as I've already mentioned, have fascinated and excited me since I was a small boy. I expect that surprises you; John Brennan, the lad in the suit who hangs out with his colourful big brother and can tell you where the dessert spoon is meant to go, doesn't seem like the kind of person who would love large, noisy, petrol-guzzling machines, does he? Well, here's something you didn't know: because I love bikes, and the bigger and noisier they are, the better.

It's hard for me to tell you exactly what it is about them I admire, because I think it's fair to say I'm entranced by every aspect of them. I love their lines, which manage to be both sleek and aerodynamic while also speaking of power and force. I adore the colours, which often combine the bright splash of primary reds and blues with the metallic of chrome and silver. I feel a thrill at the sound of a bike as it thunders past, that roar and boom when it whooshes by, and if you're on the footpath you can actually feel the air being pushed aside as the bike rips through on its way to God knows where.

Bikes speak to me in a way a lot of other things don't. Somehow, I understand them, and when I was ten years old, I decided I was going to learn everything I could about these gorgeous feats of engineering. By the time I was 11, I could name every bike I saw as I went about town, not to mention countless models I would never see in real life. Despite my difficulty at reading at school, I read every word I could find on my specialist subject and developed the ability to find even a tiny reference to any bike that caught my interest among the countless back issues of magazines I now owned.

It's a bizarre truth about my particular learning difficulty that while I struggled to make my way through a page of a book or a newspaper, I could absorb the tiniest and most obscure piece of information in a bike magazine, even those with the most spidery print you could imagine. I sat up late into the night examining diagrams and images of new models, and could tell you every single part of each one and where it was meant to go. Horsepower, braking distance, engine capacity – all these details were at the tip of my tongue. And I wasn't blinkered by the big sellers like Honda, Yamaha or Suzuki. I gravitated to the Laverda, Moto Guzzi and Ducati brands, as I loved their cutting-edge design.

Yet no one I knew owned a bike, and if I'm honest, I never really saw myself owning one either. I always knew they were dangerous, and just couldn't imagine myself kitted out in leather astride a Harley or a Honda.

So why the obsession? That's not easy to answer either. I'm a big music fan, and bikes have always had a place in the heart of rock musicians, and that's probably part of what first got me interested. I watched TV like any kid growing up in the 1970s, and of course bikers were portrayed as a little bit dangerous and wild, and as deeply mysterious and interesting. And for a middle-class kid growing up in the grey and drab world of Ireland in the seventies – a grim time to grow up in Ireland if ever there was one – that was attractive for sure.

Maybe the inner rebel in me, which is never all that deeply below the surface, was drawn to a hobby that slightly alarmed the adults in my life. I can't really negate that as a possibility, because, as someone with a long history of adventures in the world of business behind me, I know that rebellious nature is very much a part of my makeup.

But I think the real reason for my interest is something else entirely – something a bit more complicated. I lived in a world dominated by school, and while I didn't mind going, I was always conscious of the fact that school was a place where I didn't excel. The letters and numbers and thought processes I was supposed to adopt as signposts to knowledge appeared to me as twisted and unrecognisable, so the whole purpose of attending was lost on me. The way my teachers and the establishment they represented wanted me to learn didn't make sense, but motorbikes did.

After I moved to Sligo I had some friends who lived just up the road, the McDaniels, who had a few Honda 50s, which were fun, but seemed very boring and mundane to me – they weren't Ducatis or Moto Guzzis, works of art in their own right.

In Dublin, I would head off to school with a schoolbag that had a few textbooks at the top, but the majority of the space below packed full of magazines about my mechanical passion. I know my teachers would never have approved, but I still don't feel guilty about it. Motorbikes got me through what could have been a difficult time, giving me a focus and empowering me, and for that I'm grateful.

Funny to say, as an adult I have still never owned a bike, though I remain very interested in them. These days, I do have a hankering for a BMW R1800, but not to ride. I'd like to hang it on the wall or park it in the corner of a room as a piece of art. That's how beautiful I think bikes are.

How One Good Teacher Changed my Life

The assistance my mother had been praying for came in the form of a new schoolteacher from West Cork. Looking back now, I realise he and I were a bit alike – for a country boy coming to teach in such a suburban school, he, too, was a fish out of water. And perhaps that is what connected us. Whatever it was, after a couple of weeks of gentle coaxing, all of which failed, he looked me in the eye, pulled on the bit of a beard he had, and something clicked. For the first time in my schooling – I was by this time about eight years old – a teacher really saw me. And I want to stress the importance of that word: teacher.

Finbarr O'Driscoll was a teacher as opposed to someone who simply delivered the curriculum. He was interested, committed, and clearly viewed teaching as the art of connecting with the young people who populated his classroom, as opposed to force-feeding them standardised lessons laid down by the Department of Education.

I loved him and want to stress that without his help and support, nothing that follows in this story could have happened. To put it plainly, Finbarr O'Driscoll made it possible for me to have the life I have, and for that I am eternally grateful.

The first step to finding out how to help me learn was identifying the type of supports I needed. Finbarr instinctively knew I required assistance that was just not available in mainstream schools in the 1970s, and after much consultation with my mother, he arranged for an assessment with a specialist in Lad Lane in Dublin.

So off I went one Saturday morning, resplendent in tweed shorts, shirt, tie, sleeveless sweater and jacket, travelling on the Number 44 bus, hand in hand with my mother. I cannot remember the name of the educational psychologist who carried out my assessment, but I do recall he was American, and seemed very pleasant. His office was dominated by a fine antique desk and two matching chairs, which even as a young boy I understood were supposed to let me know this kind-faced man and I were on the same level – equals. He took out a piece of A4 paper and asked me to spell the word *bed*.

I remember freezing. Such a simple request. I knew it was a small, short word, one that any of my friends at school could write without a moment's thought. I even knew it started with the letter 'b', but after that I was lost. I gazed at the sheet of paper, and then at the man seated across from me, expecting to see that look of vexation and disappointment I was becoming so used to.

To my surprise, it wasn't there. Instead, I saw empathy and compassion in the American's pale-blue eyes. He was so considerate that for the first time when faced with the reality of my learning difficulties, I didn't feel embarrassed or intimidated. 'Okay,' he said, speaking in a calm and friendly voice. 'Think about a bed for a moment. What does it look like? Well, it has a headboard at the top, a flat bit in the middle, and a kicker at the end.' I'd never heard the term 'kicker' before – I later learned it's an American word – but I knew right away what he meant.

And as he said those words, my mind conjured up first a picture of a bed, then the letters 'b' and 'd'. With a little prompting, I finally put an 'e' in the middle, to represent that 'flat bit'. It was simple, visual and fun to learn. And before I left the office, I learned something else important. I wasn't naughty, I wasn't stupid and I wasn't lazy. I had a condition many successful and very intelligent people live with, it's just not the norm but that is alright and perhaps even better. Unfortunately, it had a name most of the people it afflicts struggle to pronounce, let alone write down, but at least I knew what was up with me, and I secretly thought it sounded exotic. I bounced out the door to a nervous mother, delighted to report I had a 'condition' called dyslexia, but please, please don't ask me to spell it.

Finbarr took special interest in me after that. I went to summer school in Bray for three weeks every summer and attended a few classes there during the winter. It was a different world and offered me a new lens through which I could see myself and how I responded to the challenges I faced every day. Most importantly though, it taught me that I was not – and am not – alone. I met lots of other young people who dealt with the exact same problems I did, and just knowing that made me feel less isolated and lonely.

It's important to note here that, even after all this help and support from the age of seven, I am still not a reader and spelling remains a genuine effort. But very few people know, as I have developed techniques for dealing with it. There are many ways to express oneself, and I see my shortcomings in the field of literacy as an opportunity to explore these alternative ways of communicating. For example, I regularly find myself so flummoxed by a word that even Bill Gates and his wonderful spell-checking software is unable to point me in the right direction. Perhaps he isn't the genius people think he is after all or God forbid, has dyslexia!

When this happens, the only sensible thing to do is to change direction altogether, so pause, think about the meaning I'm trying to convey, and come up with a sentence that says the same thing in a different way. This has happened umpteen times writing this book. At this stage I do it without even realising I'm doing it – although I would love to have a chat with Bill Gates about ways of improving his spell check program!

Dyslexia – What Exactly are we Talking About?

I suppose I should explain to you exactly what dyslexia is, because there are a lot of misapprehensions about it, mostly based on how it's portrayed in films and on television. When I was first diagnosed, I'd never heard of it before; most people in Ireland probably hadn't either. But these days it's much more widely known, if only partially understood.

Dyslexia is classified as a learning disorder that involves difficulty reading. This difficulty is rooted in problems identifying speech sounds and learning how they relate to letters and words, a process known to psychologists and speech therapists as decoding. If you stop and think about it, language and reading are complicated things. We look at the world around us, full of people and places and animals and plants and buildings and furniture and machines, and for each of these things, we create a sound that we use to signify that thing. Then at a particular stage in every child's development, they recognise that when Mum or Dad makes that noise, they are speaking about that animal or person or thing. Dyslexic people can do that reasonably well, although they do sometimes have problems retaining the information, and complicated words made up of lots of different sounds can be a real challenge. But they usually get them in the end.

The next part of the process is where the real problems

begin. You see, people want to be able to record their thoughts and feelings, and this is done through the written word (although with the popularity of audiobooks and speech-to-text software, this is getting a bit easier).

Writing requires coming to terms with an alphabet, each letter of which makes a different sound, and you need to know how all those squiggly symbols interact with one another. When an 'h' is beside an 's', that makes them behave differently than when they're on their own, for example. And there are rules about how they are ordered, and these rules all have exceptions, and so on and so forth. Letters come together to create written words, which then represent the sounds we use to speak about the animals, people and things I've already mentioned.

And this is where the decoding problems occur. Dyslexia affects the area of the brain that processes language recognition. The neural pathways don't work the same way they do in other people, so dyslexics need to develop different ways of coping – they need to reprogramme their thought processes. As a result they have distinct ways of learning, of which visualisation is a big part – headboard, flat bit in the middle and kicker.

People with dyslexia have normal intelligence and usually possess normal vision and hearing, although parents and teachers can often wonder if these kids are deaf, because they can have difficulty processing spoken information, particularly complicated lists of things – it's that decoding again, it just takes longer to sort out what you're being told.

There's no cure for dyslexia. Let me get that out of the way right now. Early assessment and intervention are essential, and if you can get your child the support they need, there's no reason whatsoever that they can't achieve anything any other child can. The path they take to get there might be a little different, but that's a big part of the message I want to communicate in this book. Education comes in all shapes and forms.

So what are the symptoms then? How can you tell if your child might need an assessment? Before I get into this, I need to issue a disclaimer: I don't want anyone reading this to worry or start believing their child has problems they don't, and I'm not pretending to be an educational expert, so please take these as a simple yardstick. What follows in this chapter is intended to demystify what could seem like a strange and frightening condition, but in fact is one that really isn't anything to be scared of. So let's have a look at what is involved.

Signs of dyslexia can be difficult to recognise before a child starts attending school, but a few early signs may indicate your child needs to be taught a little differently from other children their age. Some children with dyslexia are late starting to talk, and they may learn new words slowly. Others have difficulty forming words correctly – they'll reverse the sounds, for instance, or they might confuse two words that sound alike. Obviously, there will be problems remembering or naming letters, numbers and colours, and most dyslexic children will struggle to learn nursery rhymes or play rhyming games. In fact, they may show no interest in those activities at all. I certainly didn't – I distinctly remember thinking, 'What's the point in learning that?'

For children like that, the key is keeping those games

simple and straightforward, and adding visual cues to help with retention. For example, take a rhyme like this one:

I'm a little teapot, short and stout.
Here's my handle and here's my spout.
When the tea is ready, hear me shout:
Pick me up and pour me out.

The rhyme is short, only four lines, and each line contains short and simple words. But even better, it has actions that go along with it, so the child can visualise the lines which helps to remember them.

Once your child starts school, symptoms of dyslexia will become more obvious. Speaking from experience, I struggled with my letters right from the first day. Dyslexic children will read well below the expected level for their age, and they will also have problems processing and understanding what they hear. This is why undiagnosed children are often mistaken as being wilful or disobedient. But what might appear as bad behaviour is, in fact, down to the child just not understanding what they've been asked to do.

School-going dyslexic children can also be incorrectly seen as having lower intelligence, often because they seem to be constantly getting answers wrong. The reality is they may know the answer, but have difficulty finding the right word and therefore cannot form the response to the question they've been asked. What they need is more time.

Sequencing is another struggle. Doing things like maths problems can be a nightmare, because remembering you have to do this first, then that, then the other thing can be very challenging for some people who live with dyslexia. These days children with a diagnosis are given extra time to do tests and exams, and can even access people to read exam papers for them, and help them break down the questions into more easy-to-understand chunks, which is a great improvement.

And then there's all the problems with the simple task of reading, which almost everything in school is based around. For a dyslexic child there will be huge difficulty seeing (and occasionally hearing) similarities and differences in letters and words; they will have a complete inability to sound out the pronunciation of an unfamiliar word; they will struggle to spell even the simplest of words (like 'bed'), and they will spend an unusually long time completing tasks that involve reading or writing. All this means they will do their utmost to avoid such activities, even if that means acting out so they'll be sent to the bold corner. Teachers need to understand this – patience, sensitivity and emotional support are all critical at this stage.

With our increased understanding of dyslexia, children are being diagnosed early, but there are still some who slip through the net and arrive in secondary school without ever having received help or support. Teens will exhibit all the symptoms I've mentioned, but some other signs could be trouble understanding jokes or expressions that have a meaning not easily understood from the specific words. An example might be something like 'piece of cake' meaning 'easy': who thought of that, because it makes no sense!

When you are speaking to someone with very severe dyslexia, you always need to keep that in mind. There is nothing worse than being with a group of people and feeling you're being excluded from the joke. Once again, a little sensitivity goes a long way.

Dyslexic teens might have difficulty summarising a story and will struggle desperately to learn a foreign language – coping with one language is challenge enough for them! Memorising things like passages of Shakespeare or long poems will be almost impossible, and areas of maths like algebra will pose all kinds of problems.

Yet don't think this means your child can't cope with figures. I can look at a project, sum up what needs doing, and work out, usually within a very tight margin, how much it's going to cost in a flash. I might be 5 per cent out one side or the other, but I can tell you pretty accurately what the bottom line is going to be. Don't ask me to look at a spreadsheet of figures, as it'll make no sense to me, but I will know before I sit down with my accountant what he'll spend 20 minutes telling me. My mind works differently, but I get there, often much faster than a lot of other people.

Dyslexia requires fresh ways of communicating, and means you have no choice but to think outside the box. But it absolutely does not mean your child can't be the best at whatever it is they choose to do. Let them discover what that is and let them follow the path they are most comfortable with to get there. And if that path doesn't lead to a university, don't be too anxious about it. I never attended one. There are many other ways to receive an education.

Spelling Tests

'm going to jump forward in time for a moment, because this story illustrates exactly what I'm talking about. Many years after my assessment on Lad Lane I gave a job of Assistant Manager to a young Kenmare lad named Patrick Hanley. Poor Patrick spent the first few weeks at the Park in a state of constant terror, because during the week he arrived to the office I was in the middle of preparing a report for a committee I was involved with. For some this would be a quiet business, with them locked away in their office, gently typing out their thoughts and no one much the wiser about it. Not me. I would be pounding away, slowly putting my ideas on the screen in front of me when all of a sudden I would come to a word I – or the machine – could not spell. Usually I would try a few configurations to see if I could work it out, but more often than not the problem would get the better of me. As I said, Microsoft's spell check program is not always the dyslexic's best friend.

When this happened, there was only one course of action open to me. Turning in my chair, I would shout the offending word to the receptionist on duty, who would promptly spell it out to me (just as loudly) so I could keep typing. It was a ritual that would happen maybe four times a day without any discussion. The staff was well used to it by then, and everyone just got on with it. We're a family at the Park, and while it was well known I struggle with literacy, no one ever made a big deal out of it or made me feel uncomfortable.

Once the word had been spelled out, I would generally reply, 'That's a funny little word' (which it rarely was, but to me, the way the English language is written is an ongoing voyage of discovery), and my receptionist would kindly agree: 'Oh, it's a strange word alright, John,' even if it was the third or fourth time they'd spelled that same word for me that day.

There are some words that get me each and every time, no matter how many times I have to write them. Take 'library' for example. My dyslexic mind tells me to spell the word we use to describe a building where people go to borrow books like this: *libury*. When I put that into Microsoft Word, a red line appears underneath it, informing me I've spelt it incorrectly.

So I click on 'Spelling and Grammar'. The way this piece of software works is to offer the person writing the document a series of suggestions as to the word they are trying to spell. If you put in *libury*, the word it suggests you want is *liberty*, which is of course not what I'm looking for, and anyway, is a word I can spell instantly if called upon to do so, which I rarely am.

When this happens, I shout out *libury* and the receptionist comes to my rescue, and if there's no receptionist about or I'm working from home on my own, I simply Google *book libury* and hey presto, up comes *Do you mean book library*?

The week poor Patrick joined us at the Park, though, there was lots of shouting going on. Many years later, that same young man and I were involved in striking a deal to open 600 bedrooms in Dublin 4. It was a challenging and fraught negotiation that involved many late nights, and Patrick and I worked very closely together.

That kind of environment fosters close friendships, and one night he and I were having a glass of wine after a tiring day, and were reminiscing about days gone by when he suddenly said to me:

'John, do you remember when I started at the Park? That very first week?'

'I remember it well,' I told him. 'I wasn't sure you'd make it – you seemed to be terrified of your own shadow.'

'It wasn't my shadow I was afraid of,' he laughed. 'It was you who scared me!'

That floored me, because I like to think of myself as very approachable.

'Why were you scared of me? I mean, I noticed you were a ball of nerves, always running out of the office for reasons best known to yourself.'

'I ran out every time you shouted!' he said.

That really puzzled me, because I'm not a shouter, by any means. I never have been. As far as I'm concerned, courtesy costs nothing.

'I don't remember ever shouting at you, Patrick,' I said.

'No, I don't mean you were giving out to me,' he laughed. 'I thought you were giving the staff spelling tests! I was there a week before I copped you weren't.'

That made me laugh my head off. He simply hadn't been there for long enough to know how I shouted at the receptionist for help with my spelling, and how they shouted back at me, quite amicably.

Starting a Libury

B ack in that Balally primary school my education continued. I gradually improved but was always in the lower 10 per cent of the class. Any illusions I might have had that the help I was now getting from the special classes on a Saturday would turn me into a Rhodes Scholar rapidly vanished. But that was okay, as I never particularly wanted to be an academic anyway and the small improvement made the process of schooling a bit more bearable.

Sport was not my thing either, although I gave it a good try. I played everything: soccer, tennis, racquet ball, even bingo on Thursday nights in the parish hall. But I never felt inclined to join a team or to go out and play football or hurling on Saturday mornings.

Other things were beginning to attract my interest. I didn't know it at the time, but the world of business and the excitement of creating businesses or ideas was starting to call out to me. And in a peculiar twist of fate, it was books that formed the basis of my very first entrepreneurial venture.

I'd caught one of those bugs small children tend to get, and the doctor informed my mother I needed to be off school for at least a week. The first couple of days I was so ill I didn't much care where I was, and just lay in bed feeling sorry for myself. On the third or fourth day, however, I started to rally, and pretty soon boredom set in. What could I do to pass the time? I paced the room like a caged tiger – albeit one in Sesame Street pyjamas – and finally my eyes fell onto the pile of books my mother had left on my bedside locker in the hopes I might feel inspired to open one during my convalescence.

I sat on the edge of the bed and looked at the tower of children's stories. There was a Doctor Seuss and a couple of Noddy books. A collection of fairy tales and a colourful picture book all about trucks and tractors (which was the only one I'd even opened).

Suddenly, the seed of an idea took root in my head, and over the next hour it started to blossom, and then to bloom. That's how it is with me. I can see a concept grow and flourish as I tease it out and shape it. Sometimes it becomes a beautiful, strong tree; other times a gorgeous flower. Occasionally it's one of those tall cactuses like you see in the westerns or the cover of a U2 album. But once it has a form, I know I'm onto something and it generally gets put into action very quickly.

This idea was about how I could make those books, which I habitually saw as utterly useless, actually be of benefit to me. Our house was full of books of all kinds. My mother liked romance and crime novels. My father read adventure stories and thrillers set in Africa and other far-flung, exotic climes. Damien had a collection of spiritual writings and Christian apologetics, as well as a fine bunch of Louis L'Amour cattle operas. My sisters enjoyed Jane Austen and historical novels, and there were loads of cookbooks and DIY manuals, not to mention plenty of encyclopaedias and reference texts too. In other words, all tastes were catered for.

I remember sitting on the windowsill in my bedroom, looking out on the road, and all I could see were housewives and homemakers all heading to do their shopping in H. Williams, the large supermarket that had recently opened at the end of our road. I could also spy a couple of bus stops at which crowds of people were gathered, many reading newspapers or magazines.

H. Williams had not done my father's shop any favours, and the bus stops in Stepaside whisked customers away from his door. But both served my newly hatched endeavour well by giving me that most important of resources for any fledgling business: foot traffic.

My idea was simple. H. Williams has a small rack of paperbacks that were always surrounded by women, looking for something interesting to read, but the choice they offered was limited. The people at the bus stop would surely be interested in something other than those boring novels.

At the age of seven I had identified a gap in the market, one I was determined to exploit. I decided to convert Francis's old bedroom in the garage (he had just moved to begin a job in Cork) into a library. My terms would be a little different from the standard public library system, in that my clients would pay me a rental fee for each book they took out. I even worked out a pricing system based around the number of pages, whether or not the book was a paperback or hardback, if it was illustrated or not, and so on. Children's books and educational texts were set at a cheaper rate, because they were for youngsters, and any volumes that were too wrinkled looking or had torn covers were placed in a kind of bargain bin and could be rented at rock-bottom prices.

I spent the rest of the week organising my new venture and making it as professional as possible. I labelled and categorised all the books, placing them in alphabetical order along lines of subject matter – I could recognise letters and knew to look only at the second name of the author on the spine, so this was doable for me. I created rental cards and drafted membership criteria. I decided local people should be given priority, as it would be easier to track down errant borrowers, but if a prospective client was on an easily accessed bus route, we could probably do business with them.

I couldn't wait to get started and was planning my business launch with great delight. Everything was going remarkably well and I was sure I was on to a winner when, to my dismay, the doctor returned. In the halcyon days of the 1970s house calls were still common, and in my enthusiasm, I had forgotten I was home from school sick. Regrettably, my mother saw my energetic commitment to the library project as a sign I was on the mend, and the doctor agreed. To my disgust he cleared my return to school for the following Monday.

I never got to open my library. But I never forgot it, or the excitement and happiness I found in planning and developing that seed into (almost) full maturity. At seven years of age, I was already thinking about business.

The Not-So Sporting Life

As I said in the previous chapter, sport isn't really my thing. To put that in context, I've never been to a match in Croke Park. The only time I've ever attended an event in Ireland's most celebrated sports ground was to see the rock band U2 perform. It was a great gig, and part of me thinks seeing the greatest band in the world perform in such an historic location added something to the overall experience. That said, I've seen bands play in tiny pubs in Sligo and been just as excited. In fact one such band *was* U2, who played in the Blue Lagoon in Sligo town in 1980. I was only 15 but managed to get in (age restrictions were less rigidly upheld in those days). I remember it well, as it was a Monday night and I should not have been out at all, but the staff of my brother's pub were all talk about it over the weekend, and I insisted I be brought along too.

It's a gig I won't ever forget. U2 were one of the hottest Irish bands on the circuit at the time, and while the room was crowded, loud and smoky, there was a rawness and honesty to the group's performance that was amazing to see. I feel very lucky to have been there.

As I now live in Templenoe, just outside Kenmare, we are surrounded by GAA clubs, but I never go to matches. This is not because I'm not interested, but because I seem to carry a jinx with me. As strange as this might sound, I've never been to a match where the team I was supporting won.

Recently, the lads from Templenoe's football team had a really important game, and a club member rang to invite me to attend as their guest.

'I'm awfully sorry, but I'm going to have to say no,' I told him. 'If I show up, you'll lose, and it'll be my fault, not yours.'

I hope he understood: I stayed away for their own good! I've always had conflicted feelings about sport. I both love it and hate it.

I played soccer as a kid, mostly in goal. I was good, but not great. In school I played table tennis, and was quite competent at that. As an adult I love watching the rugby and Formula 1.

But my love-hate relationship with sport doesn't mean I don't understand how important it is. Because I think the Irish attitude to sport is central to why we are such a success internationally. The Gaelic Athletic Association, that guardian of our traditional sports, hurling and Gaelic football, has instilled in us something that may appear simple but is in fact deeply complex, though it seems every child in the country understands on a cellular level.

Think about it like this: every county in Ireland has lots of local teams, all of whom play against one another for the county title. So in Kerry you'll have Kenmare Shamrocks and Templenoe and Shannon Rangers and St Kieran's, and the supporters of those teams, all of whom identify powerfully with the townlands they represent, will go to matches and see themselves in fierce competition with one another. It will be absolutely tribal and ferocious. Yet when the county team is in the All Ireland, they're all Kerry supporters, come to do battle with a rival county side.

That sense of competition, but also of unity, carries through into our national identity. I've met Irish people when I'm abroad, many of whom are working at the highest levels in the hospitality industry, operating front of house in Michelin-starred restaurants or managing five-star hotels. I've met CEOs in major companies who are proudly Irish, and I know precisely what got them there. They approached the task of working their way up through the ranks of whichever company they found themselves in with a sense of healthy competition against all others in the running for promotion, while remaining loyal to their employers. And this sets the Irish apart. That and their ability to talk to complete strangers and find common ground.

Sport and the camaraderie and fellowship it fosters teaches communication skills, the ability to forge relationships, the necessity of being a team player. And maybe most importantly, good sports people are task-oriented problem solvers. I don't want one of my managers to come to me and point out a problem. I want them to tell me there was a problem, but they solved it.

Sport teaches problem-solving and the GAA ensures it is in the DNA of every young person in the country. That is some service to the country that goes far beyond sport. If only they didn't have games and training at weekends when the hospitality industry needs all those young people at work I would be much happier! So while I'm not much of a player, I would certainly classify myself as a sports fan. And seeing a history of involvement in sports on someone's CV always piques my interest.

A Burst of Colour Makes All the Difference

When I followed in my brothers' footsteps and started secondary school in CUS, I hated it. It was academic and I wasn't. They expected me to learn Latin, but I was struggling to grasp the intricacies of English. The school sports were cricket and rugby, which were totally alien to me, and the classes were full of rich kids, some of whom were friendly but others who seemed distant and unfriendly.

The school offered me nothing I wanted, and in turn, I brought nothing but resentment and hostility to it. It was a repressed, quiet kind of hostility, and it took the form of my simply opting out. The establishment and everything it stood for left me cold, so I decided I had better just serve my time and hope no one would pay any notice. And no one did. I even hated the trappings of the place. Somehow, I felt like a total fraud in my blazer and tie. They felt wrong on me. As if I was dressed up as something opposite to who I was supposed to be.

But I always attended, never caused any outward fuss, and continued my participation in the lower 10 per cent, just about passing my end-of-year tests. I distinguished myself at nothing, but as I was left alone and the teachers didn't bother with me, the experience had little negative impact on my life.

I knew I had to go to school, and one miserable location was much the same as any other. I just put my head down and got on with it.

The highlight of each day for me was catching a glimpse of the beautiful gardens at Pye Televisions, an electronics firm that was based where the new Dundrum Town Centre is now. Most people didn't even know these gardens, which were ornamental wonders, even existed, but just at the point where the bus stopped to let me off, the wall was low enough to get a really good view if you were on the upper deck. I would stand on tiptoe and crane my neck, basking in the explosion of colour from the beautifully laid out flower beds and deeply inhaling the scent of pollen. It was like seeing a panoramic view of paradise before being forced to enter purgatory, and I would drink it in before running down the spiral stairs to get off the bus.

That single brief snatch of something bright and perfect kept me going through my decidedly imperfect days. And it taught me a lesson. A break from the norm, even a short one like feasting my eyes on those beautiful gardens, can revive the soul.

Tom Brennan – My Dad the Shopkeeper

I f I sit for a moment and close my eyes, I can picture my dad very clearly. He was always dapper, and wore a crisp white shirt with a tie, always of a strong colour, though rarely patterned. This would be matched with a jumper or cardigan, occasionally what we would today call a sports jacket, and slacks with a sharp crease ironed into them. His shoes always gleamed, and his hair always looked freshly barbered and perfectly held in place with oil and pomade. And there would, more often than not, be a cigarette smouldering in his hand.

Tom Brennan was a teetotaller – he took the pledge never to drink alcohol at his confirmation and kept it his entire life – but he smoked whatever he could lay his hands on. His cigarette of choice was Carroll's non-filter, but my mother always said he would smoke brown paper if nothing else was available.

I never thought anything of it, as everyone smoked at the time. My mother always had her cigarette attached to one of those long cigarette holders, which I thought made her look extremely sophisticated. It also meant the tobacco never stained her fingers. I remember my dad used to wash his hands constantly to make sure they never had that yellow stain – it wouldn't do for a shopkeeper to be seen as anything other than impeccably turned out.

And this followed through in how he ran his business. Dad's shop was never less than perfect. All the labels faced outwards, so you only had to glance at the product to know what it was. The shelves were stocked to the front for ease of access. The place was gleaming and spotless, and even had a customer toilet when such things were virtually unheard of – my dad had heard about such a convenience from someone, and decided his store had to have one.

My dad was a man of ideas. A man who wanted to get things done. He was always dreaming up ways of making his shop bigger and better and more attractive to his group of loyal customers. Even as a kid I admired his tenacity and dedication. My father had a powerful work ethic, and he passed it on to all of his children, just as it had been passed down to him.

Dad's father, my grandad, worked with the Office of Public Works. A lover of gardening, he was a gifted woodworker who could tease beautiful things from pieces of oak and ash. Thankfully, we still have many pieces of his creation in the family. His life ended far too early as a result of a weak chest but there is a rose named after him in the Botanic Gardens, the Brennan Rose, which is a nice thing to have.

I believe my father's affinity for the world of business, though, was inspired by his mother. Qualities like resilience, problem solving, thrift and dedication were instilled in him from a young age by this titan of a woman.

Granny Brennan was widowed at the young age of 34, and despite remarkable adversity she raised four children, owned and ran two shops and many houses in the Milltown area – by no means an easy task for a widowed mother in the

Ireland of the 1940s. Dad had that mettle in his bones, and as soon as he was old enough, he determined to go out on his own, buying the shop in Stepaside.

That little shop was his pride and joy, and it showed in the love he lavished on it and in his attention to detail. It was also obvious in how he treated the people he worked alongside and those he served. Many of his staff and countless former customers remained in contact with my mother until the day she died, and this left a huge impression on me: it taught me that business is a human endeavour. Although money is important, success does not have to be measured by how much money you make. It can also be measured in the quality of the relationships you form, and the impact you have on the lives of the people you meet along the way.

My father taught me how to do things well. His philosophy was that, if a job is worth doing, you should give it 100 per cent of your love and attention. Anything less was simply not good enough. I didn't know it at the time, but I learned more from him in the short time I spent helping out in the shop than I did in many full-time jobs I was to occupy.

I think the biggest lesson, and the one that I try to impart to my own staff, is that the difference between doing something right and getting it wrong is very little. Sometimes it's a minuscule mistake, but the fallout can be vast. For example, Dad's shop was located just past the famous Stepaside Garda Station, and one of the bus stops I've already mentioned was located right outside the front door. This was a source of constant business, because when the people living in St Patrick's Estate nearby got off the bus, they regularly popped in for a bar of chocolate or a bag of sweets to bring home to their kids. It meant there was a constant flow of trade, and all that chocolate and sweets added up to a reasonable profit margin at the end of the week, although we were never going to get rich from it.

At some stage, though, the bus stop was moved 100 metres up the road in a bid to alleviate a traffic bottleneck, and all that business ceased. Such a small thing in the mind of the urban planner, but it had a colossal impact on my father's business and on the Brennans as a family.

Dad always had an Opel Rekord estate. It doubled as a family car and a delivery vehicle. At this time Feargal Quinn was still to bring the concept of the supermarket to Ireland, so my father's type of shop was where people went for groceries before continuing on to their local butcher, then the baker and so on – very different from the way people shop today. It meant that entire communities relied on the shops that served them, socialising in them, getting the local news and gossip, and experiencing important human contact. In those days you really *knew* the person who served you your bread or your pound of sausages, and they in turn knew you, and were concerned about your welfare. If a customer was elderly and couldn't carry their groceries home, Dad would pop them into the Opel, and make sure they arrived at their destination in time for dinner. That was my dad. Neat. Attentive. Reliable. Good hearted. And that personality permeated through to the shop he loved so dearly.

Unfortunately, it all came to an end far too soon. But let me share a happy memory with you before I get to that. Let me tell you about my earliest memories of the hospitality industry. About the first time I ate out in a posh restaurant.

Days at the Beach and Having Someone at My Service

D ad closed the shop at 1 p.m. on Monday afternoons, which meant that during the summer, the family could enjoy trips to Brittas Bay, a gorgeous beach in County Wicklow. Those Monday afternoons were special. I would sit in the class bobbing up and down like a rabbit, peering out the window to see if that big estate car was at the gate. Brittas Bay meant sandcastles, swimming in the sea, sandy banana sandwiches (for some reason my mother always used to mash the bananas, which I still hate) and just tremendous fun.

There was nothing fancy or contrived about those sunny trips to the sea. They were simple but *real*. My parents lavished their time and their love on us, and built lasting memories that I still treasure. I think what made them so special was the fact that Dad worked so hard. He never had a holiday in the true sense, perhaps a couple of days here and another day there, but these were often broken by some emergency that had him rushing back to the shop.

Self-employed people give up so much, and that was especially true back then. There was no pension, no dole, no insurance and virtually no support from the government. It was an extraordinarily difficult lifestyle, and those Mondays were his only release.

Forget golf. Forget junkets to shopkeepers' conferences in the Shelbourne. He worked long hours because that was what was required to keep his family fed, clothed and educated. End of story. He didn't drink, he wasn't a sports fan and he didn't go to concerts or plays. Those days at the beach were his way of relaxing, and when I recollect them now, I always see him with a smile on his face. On the way back home, if business had been good the week before, we would be asked a question.

'The La Touche in Greystones or Beaufield Mews in Stillorgan for dinner?'

And therein lies a story – a tale of two restaurants. Because although we had very little in way of wealth, Mum and Dad knew style and liked the occasional brush with luxury. They would never go to a pub or go out to dinner as a couple, but they loved bringing us to nice places on rare occasions as opposed to mediocre places regularly. It was a subtle lesson for the five of us, one that has cost us all a fortune but has also made our lives worth living.

When I think of the La Touche, there's one thing that always comes to mind immediately. Their chips. The La Touche had the best chips I have ever tasted. They were small and crispy and I can still recall how delicious they were. Taste memory is extremely powerful, and the best chefs know how to manipulate that and transport a diner to a favourite place or a specific childhood moment. The chef in La Touche was a genius, because it is that *taste* I remember vividly. Whatever oil he used was light and subtle, leaving a golden chip with enough fluffy potato inside to be a proper, hearty bite. I can attest that a chip of this quality is extremely hard to find. And I know because I have spent the rest of my life looking.

The dining room of the restaurant was posh but not stuffy and overlooked the ocean. I remember crisp white tablecloths, stemmed glasses and deep pile carpet, which all added to the experience. We may have only gone ten times over as many summers, but it was magical, and we knew it was a treat. And most importantly, it was a lesson in how to create an experience that resonated. One I never forgot.

When business was *really* good we went to The Beaufield Mews. This was posh, probably a little bit prim, but I thought it was pure class. The room sparkled with crystal, you draped linen napkins across your knees, and your order was taken by the maître d'. Whatever you were drinking, one of the waiting staff poured it for you.

And the food. Well, it was special, and like nothing I'd had before. They served a veal Milanese, cooked tableside and served from the left. I was probably about seven or eight and this was something very few kids my age would have experienced. As opposed to the gorgeous chips of La Touche, Beaufield Mews had hand-turned roast potatoes cooked in goose fat and sprinkled with sea salt, aromatic with roast thyme. I could not get enough of them. I know what you're thinking: how very Irish that the two foods I most remember, and still crave, are both potato-based. And I'm not going to apologise for it.

These two restaurants taught me a life's lesson: if you can get the simple things right, everything else will follow.

How Your Life Can Turn Upside-down Overnight

My father seemed to become ill overnight, his beloved cigarettes winning in the end, as they often do. The strange and terrible thing is that none of us saw it coming. He seemed to be perfectly healthy, doing all the things he always did with all the enthusiasm he always had on the Friday, and then on the Saturday: boom! Everything was different and our world was never the same again.

I have learned that monumental change can happen in a second. This is a fundamental truth in business, but in the world of checks and balances and negotiations and deals, there is almost always something you can do to turn a disaster around. I have pulled sinking ships back from the brink of annihilation more times than I care to remember.

But with Dad, the damage had been done. Those weak lungs that took his father at such a young age were a legacy he couldn't avoid, and his lifelong love of tobacco took its toll, a toll he had no option but to pay. My father collapsed behind the counter of his treasured shop in Stepaside one Saturday afternoon. One moment he was upright, serving customers and chatting as always, the next he was on the floor, grey, haggard and gasping for breath. He was sixty years old – still a young man, by today's standards.

The terrible thing is I'm sure he *wasn't* okay in the days and weeks running up to his collapse. I have a feeling he was probably suffering, but as was his way, chose to soldier on and not worry any of us about it. Men aren't good at talking about their health even in these more enlightened times, but in the 1970s, suffering in silence was just the way it was done – until it got so bad he couldn't function anymore.

My father spent three weeks in the intensive care unit (ICU) in St Vincent's Hospital, and those three weeks were some of the most stressful and upsetting my family ever experienced. Mum tried to protect us from it, but she couldn't. The anxiety was writ large across her face. It was touch and go many times during those terrible days, and Dad received the Sacrament of the Anointing of the Sick twice. For those of you who aren't au fait with the various sacraments of the Roman Catholic Church, the Anointing of the Sick takes place when a person is near death, so that tells you how bad things were. Effectively, they thought my father was going to die on at least two occasions.

That's what my mother was trying to carry alone. We rallied around and I tried to give her all the love and support I could, but I was only 11 years old, and was probably more scared than she was. Yet Tom Brennan fought his way back. The skills of the medical team combined with his inbuilt resilience and the powerful love he had for his family brought my dad back from the brink.

After he left the ICU, he spent a further three weeks in hospital, and we learned that his lungs were now operating on only a small percentage of their full capacity. My father would be dependent on oxygen for the rest of his life and would never be able to do many of the things he – and indeed *we* – had taken for granted. In the space of a very small period of time, our family life changed irrevocably.

I didn't know it then, but the events of that Saturday in Stepaside set me on the path I'm still following. And the first part of that journey was to bring me through some woods filled with holly trees. But before I get to that, let me tell you about how Francis tried to save my father's shop.

Brennan and Son

The Sunday after my dad collapsed was the first day
in the history of Brennan's shop in Stepaside that the
place didn't open.

This meant two things. Firstly (and let's not beat around
the bush, this is the most important point of the two) there
was no money coming in. For an independent trader, losing
a day of trading is a massive blow. Secondly, the shop being
closed left a huge hole in the community. As I've already
explained, my dad's store was a lifeline for so many people,
and its absence was felt profoundly.

Luckily, the shop didn't stay closed for long. Dad employed
a few people to help out, but none of them ever did the
crucial things like stock-taking, filling out orders, balancing
the accounts, lodging the takings – in other words, all the
critical actions needed to keep a business running smoothly.

Someone had to carry out those tasks, and we had a family
meeting to discuss how it was to be done. After much debate,
it was decided such a significant role should be kept within
the family, so Francis was chosen to return from working in
Jurys in Sligo, where he was on a college placement, to run
the shop.

I genuinely believe my older brother did this with an open
heart and the best of intentions, wanting to do the right thing
by his family and make a positive mark on the running of
Dad's business. He came bustling in with all that positive

energy Francis is so well known for, bursting with ideas and determined this was to be a new era for what was now going to be 'Brennan and Son Grocery Emporium'.

But alas, it was not to be. Francis has many skills, and I admire him greatly, but the small, precise and somewhat limited world of a local shopkeeper was never going to be the stage upon which he was destined to perform. But he gave it his all. I have to credit him with that.

My brother rearranged the layout of the products. He designed new labels for the shelves. He sat down with the staff and talked about how customers should be greeted when they came in, and developed promotions to try and sell items that weren't shifting (Dad's shop was one of those places where you could buy anything from a candle to a Swiss Army knife, which meant there were more than a few pieces of stock that had been sitting on shelves in the storage room for years). But there was always something missing during Francis's tenure.

Dad just had a way about him. For example, if the shop was empty and an old lady came in, he would spend twenty minutes chatting about something her cat did the night before, or about the latest episode of *The Riordans*, a popular Irish TV soap opera at the time. Francis is an Olympic-level talker, but his focus on the nuts and bolts of a business and his desire to be involved in every aspect of its running means that, while he's talking to Mrs Boyle about her new bird feeder, he's also thinking about a pallet of tinned beans that need unpacking out the back and wondering if the young fella he tasked with the job is doing it right.

In a large hotel, there are other people to take care of all of this. In a small shop, he felt a weight of responsibility. He knew talking to the customers and lavishing them with attention was important, but when he was nattering, he felt guilty that he wasn't doing the hundred and one other things he had on the copious lists he compiled every morning over his breakfast.

Francis held the show together for a heroic five months, but in the end it was clear to anyone who knew him that my big brother was absolutely miserable. If there was ever a man who is built to work in the hotel business, it's Francis Brennan. It is simply the way he is designed. He breathes, eats and sleeps hotels. Keeping him from his great love was an act of cruelty, and my father and mother both recognised this, and in a show of remarkable parental kindness, they released Francis from the obligation he felt he owed them.

Brennan and Son Grocery Emporium was sold. Francis returned to Sligo, and I went for that walk in the woods. It was to be a very important stroll indeed.

Christmas Logs and a Lesson in Costing

Dad was discharged from hospital, but he needed supplemental oxygen for fifteen hours out of every day for the rest of his life.

Where before he was rarely seen without a cigarette between the thumb and forefinger of his right hand, now he was distinguished by the oxygen machine he needed to be connected to, and the long tube with cannulas that fed the life-giving vapour into his nostrils.

With time on his hands for the first time in his life, my father bought a shed for the back garden and, drawing on his father's accomplishments, began to dabble in woodwork, making shadow boxes, a few ornaments and some other oddments. While he didn't have his father's flair or natural ability, he was more than competent, and the items he produced were solid and well made. Sadly, his compromised lung capacity – which basically meant he couldn't process the oxygen from the air when he took it into his lungs – made working with his hands difficult, and he could never stay in his shed for very long before needing to rest.

I found that shed fascinating, though. I remember he had a drill with lots of interesting-looking bits, a jigsaw, a powerful-looking chainsaw and hammers of various shapes and sizes, all hung in dedicated places on the wall. To my chagrin, I was not allowed inside this chamber of creativity, although I did sneak longing glances in through the door when he wasn't looking. But all that was to change due to the only bit of the grocery business my father held onto.

Dad had a contract with the Catholic Boy Scouts of Ireland, supplying them with groceries at their camping grounds of Larch Hill, a tract of land in the Dublin mountains where they hosted events for the various scout clubs around the country. After he sold the shop, he held onto the contract as a modest means of income to keep us in bread and butter. Scout troops from all over the world also came to use the facility. It was a beautiful landscape of woods, leafy paths and a river that doubled as a swimming pool when the weather permitted, created by placing a sheet of wood at the narrowest end of the stream. In the centre of this wilderness were acres of flat green fields where tents could be pitched.

I always thought it a mystical place. You would pass through high white gates and, as they closed behind you, you somehow knew you were somewhere different.

I was delighted when I learned that Dad had held onto the contract with the scouts. Which meant that on quite a few Saturdays he and I would climb into the Opel, head off to the wholesalers and fill the generous boot with tins of beans and loaves of bread and all the other things a large gang of youngsters on a camping expedition might need.

One Saturday – it was during the autumn – we had just completed a delivery to Larch Hill and he and I were walking back to the Opel. Since his collapse, my dad always moved with deliberate purpose. I was getting used to this slower version of him – after just a few months I barely noticed the oxygen tank anymore – but the reduced speed with which he did everything was harder to ignore.

He stopped for a moment, looking about him at the dense foliage, listening to the sound of rooks and jackdaws chattering overhead. He paused often, now, and he'd not done that before. When I was younger he was always busy, rushing here and there. Not now. I think the pauses were partly to enjoy the world now he didn't have to be thinking about the next job or some crisis or other going on in the shop. But he was also resting. Allowing time for his damaged lungs to feed oxygen into his blood. I never drew attention to these newly initiated stops; I didn't mind them, anyway. When he paused, he talked. And I liked that.

'Do you see all those fallen branches, John?' he asked me.

I cast an eye about the woods. There were lots of large branches that had been blown down in a recent storm.

'I do,' I replied.

'And can you see that holly bush over there? And there's a couple more just a bit beyond it. These woods are full of them.'

I could easily pick out the dark-green, prickly leaves of the plant we associate with Christmas.

'And lots of the fallen branches are covered in moss. That can be dried without too much difficulty.'

That puzzled me.

'Why would you want to dry it?' I wanted to know.

'I think we should make Christmas logs,' my father said, smiling. 'You could sell them in the couple of weeks before the big day.'

I thought about it for all of 30 seconds.

'I could do that,' I said, returning his grin.

'I know you could,' he said, and that vote of confidence was all I needed.

The process of making these festive creations began in the woods of Larch Hill. Dad would drop me off, armed with a small chainsaw, and I would head into the trees and pick out windfall branches of just the right thickness. I reckoned ones with about the same circumference as a man's arm were just right. Once I had a good pile of these, I would use the chainsaw to cut them into lengths of about five feet, which would fit perfectly into the boot of the Opel (I would cut them into smaller lengths when I got home), and then pile them just off the track near those white gates, for easy loading.

I collected holly sprigs when the berries came out, which is a much narrower window of time than you might think. Here's something you may not know: only female holly bushes produce berries, and they only turn red towards the end of October and into November. You have to collect them quickly though, because those berries are a favourite food of finches, squirrels and mice. In the woods at Larch Hill, the amount of wildlife meant I had plenty of competition. Moss I harvested as I went, spreading it out on the ground near my completed bundles to ensure it started the drying process before I even brought it home.

Larch Hill provided what I thought of as the 'free' materials, although these days I would probably factor in a cost for my time investment. As an 11-year-old, though, mucking about in the woods was an adventure, and something I would happily have spent an afternoon doing anyway.

Once the woodland pieces were all transported home, I set about sourcing the other components. I knew many people would place the logs on their dinner tables, so a piece of green baize – the type of material you see covering snooker tables – would be needed on the bottom of each to prevent scratching. No log could be considered complete without a red candle, and I found out that you could purchase such items with either one-inch or half-inch diameters. Some experimentation taught me that my father's widest drill-bit could not cope with creating multiple one-inch holes, so I opted for half-inch, which I thought looked less impressive, but stopped me breaking multiple bits, which then needed to be replaced, therefore adding to our overheads.

The decoration of the logs was finished by stapling on some of the dried moss and a sprig of holly, and then I artfully sprayed each one with some artificial snow, the type you can buy in a can in novelty shops. I have to admit, the satisfaction I experienced when I stood back and surveyed my first completed Christmas log was just priceless. Now all I had to do was make hundreds more!

And I did. Dad insisted the cost of producing each log could not be more than thirty pence, and it was up to me to source the most cost-effective candles, staples, baize and spray, and to calculate precisely how much spray and staples were going to be used in the creation of each log.

For the staples that was easy: each box cost sixty pence, and there were three hundred staples in each one. This meant that each staple cost point two of a penny. If I used ten staples in a log, the overall cost of staples was two pence. The snow spray was harder. I had to work out how many sprays of a particular duration (I would push the nozzle and count 'one, two, three, four' and then stop) each can contained and then divide that into the overall cost of the can. But I got it right in the end.

It was a hugely valuable exercise and has stayed with me for life. I use the exact same technique now when I'm opening a hotel or developing any project: I work out overheads and outgoings and use that to establish how high my profit margins are likely to be. That is the most basic but important equation in any business – outgoings versus incomings. Credit versus debit. And I learned it from my father aged twelve.

It wasn't all plain sailing though. During that first year while I was refining the process, I forgot to factor in that I would need to purchase an axe. We had worked out the costings and I was more than happy with our figures, but as I started into cutting the five-foot-long logs into the smaller sizes they needed to be to be sold, I realised I would also need to split them to give them a flat bottom to sit on, so we would need an axe to do that.

I ran to tell my father I needed to buy a small hand axe – a hatchet. He looked at me patiently, and reached for his wallet, but as he handed me the money I needed he said, in tones I will never forget:

'This means your pricing is no longer accurate. You know that, don't you?'

I was furious with myself that I had made such a monumental error. So the figures could remain unaffected, I ran across the road to our neighbours, the Durhams, who I knew had the exact kind of axe I needed, and borrowed it from them. As I handed Dad back his money, he smiled.

Because he knew I had learned the lesson.

Selling the logs was easy, and I enjoyed it thoroughly. I went from house to house with Johnston Mooney and O'Brien bread trays with 12 logs on each. I made a jolly sight with my colourful, snow-sprinkled fare, and even if people didn't buy they seemed happy to see me. A lot of people did buy though, and to my surprise and delight, some asked if they could place orders for the following Christmas.

The first year of trading I sold three hundred logs, netting a profit of two hundred and ten pounds. In my second year I sold over six hundred. My dad wouldn't take a penny of the profits.

'You earned that, so it's yours to do with as you see fit,' he told me.

As a result, I had the best bike of any kid on our street. But the Christmas log project brought me much more than money. It taught me how to set up a business, and how to make it work. I now understand that this was where my education really began.

PART TWO

Going Out West

STARTING OVER

D ad's illness was not improving. The air pollution in Dublin, a combination of smoke from people's coal fires, the fumes belching out of the exhaust pipes of cars, trucks and buses and the constant fug of toxicity the factories belched skyward, was not good for the chronic bronchitis and emphysema he lived with daily.

After much deliberation and several family meetings, the decision was made to move to Sligo, where my parents built a new house right beside my mother's family farm, a place we holidayed at regularly, and somewhere I loved dearly. I was thrilled.

My time at CUS had become a slow drudge. It felt like the school and I were locked in a stalemate, a Mexican standoff which could only end badly. I really do wonder what would have become of me if I'd been forced to stay. While I had made some friends, it was a city school, so I never got to see any of them when I went home anyway, so even the process of leaving them was softened and made less traumatic.

Moving to Sligo felt like we were going home. I remember it with nothing but joy. And it wasn't just me who felt that way. My brother Damien loved the West. His calling to the priesthood had foundered and he left the seminary before ordination and moved in with our aunt and uncle, Mum's brother and sister, on the family farm.

By the time we moved west he had opened a pub called Beezies on O'Connell Street in Sligo Town. It was a big gastropub, well ahead of its time, and was already getting favourable reviews in the Irish press and rapidly becoming a very cool place to be seen when we arrived.

My sister, Susan, was also working in Sligo as a physiotherapist in Sligo General Hospital, so it felt as if the family was consolidating under Ben Bulben.

The new house was stunning: it was detached, with a tarmac drive and a large garage. A winding spiral staircase led up to my bedroom, which had a picture window overlooking Lough Gill. Downstairs there was a built-in kitchen with all the modern conveniences, and outside we enjoyed a large fenced garden with loads of lawn space and beautiful mature trees.

I remember thinking it was like something we should not own, a house you might read about in a magazine. It made me think that Sligo and the West were places dreams might come true. It turned out that I was right.

The move took place in June, so when September rolled around I had to start at a new school, something that did not fill me with much pleasure. In Sligo Town I had two choices: Summerhill or The Grammar. Neither appealed to me, as both bore unpleasant similarities to CUS. So my mother, who somehow understood on an instinctive level what was going on in my head, agreed to send me to Ballisodare, which is situated 10 miles outside Sligo Town.

On the face of it, this was a decision that made no sense and put a lot of work on Mum. With Dad being ill, she had to learn how to drive just to get around and go shopping. There was no school bus from the town to my new country school either, so I had to be driven each day, a 30-minute trip my mother made each day with stoic good humour. And I could never thank her enough for doing so, because it was the best decision she ever made. Ballisodare was the school I had been waiting for my whole young life.

The kids who attended were the sons and daughters of farmers and manual workers, and the ethos of the place was practical rather than academic. The school offered woodwork, home economics and mechanical drawing, and although they did have a sports programme, the playing field was regularly used to graze sheep, so no one was really interested in kicking a ball on it.

I settled in immediately and loved every moment of the three years I spent there. It was co-educational and run by the Mercy Nuns, a group of women who divide opinion, but I can only speak from my personal experience: I found them sensitive and extremely supportive.

Unlike at CUS, I suddenly found myself scoring in the middle of the pack at exams in a class where no one ever achieved 100 per cent and no one ever notched up 10 per cent either. It seemed a kinder, gentler, less bruising way of teaching. The classes moved at a steady pace, and rivalry and competitiveness were not encouraged. For the first time in my educational life, I felt safe and secure, and I soon made some fantastic friends, who were loyal to the last.

One of these was a young lad named Joe, who used to travel in the car with us. Mum would pick him and a couple of other kids up along the route, as she was travelling it anyway, and it meant their parents didn't have to leave their farming chores to drop them to school.

One afternoon I received a detention due to some boisterous behaviour, and my mum was ten minutes out the road for home when she noticed I was not among the group of youngsters in the back of the car.

'Where's John?' she asked, genuinely puzzled.

My pal Joe, quick on his feet, piped up:

'Oh, Mrs Brennan, don't worry yourself, he decided to walk as he was in a hurry to get home to start his homework.'

My mother, who knew better than most that this was a highly improbable story, couldn't help but laugh, as she was aware the comment stemmed not just from Joe's misplaced loyalty, but also from the fact she drove painfully slowly.

Luckily my mother's good humour prevented me receiving another punishment when I finally did arrive home. It was an early lesson in the personality and character of the people of the West.

Music: What it Means to Me

Our family home always had music, and I firmly believe that a life without music is not a life worth living. Dad loved James Last and Perry Como. My sisters liked 10cc. I desperately wanted to forge my own taste – find out what it was that spoke to me, and one day in the school yard I heard the name Bryan Ferry. For some reason it stuck with me, and I bought his new album, *The Bride Stripped Bare*, which was a decidedly racy title for a 14-year-old who attended a school run by nuns. I remember that my mother was not impressed. But I can tell you, I definitely was.

As a kid I wanted to know everything about an album when I bought it, and I still do. I'm fascinated by the sound engineer and how they achieved the tone and atmosphere of each piece. I want to know who the producer was, and their vision for the record – what they really wanted it to say.

I am particularly interested in studios, and if I love a record, I have to know what studio it was recorded in and what musicians played on each track in addition to the band. It saddens me greatly that in the world of downloads and Spotify, such gems of knowledge are no longer available. I always believe knowing these things deepens your understanding of a record. And that all began with this saucily named album.

Bryan Ferry, and music in general, remain a huge part of my life. My other hobbies I indulge in when I can, as they tend to be quite time consuming (going out on a boat, for example, requires planning and a sizeable chunk of your day), but music can be dipped into any time, and even a few moments of it are like recharging your batteries. I don't know what it is or why – I'm not a musicologist or a student of the arts, but all I can say is that songs or even instrumental pieces can move me in all kinds of ways. The sound of an acoustic guitar being strummed, the cascade of notes from a piano solo, the plaintive call of a blues harmonica, all touch me in different but profound ways.

And I've been lucky to have met and even become friends with many musicians I admire. David Gray came to stay at the Park while he was writing and rehearsing his hugely successful *White Ladder* album. As I worked in reception, I could hear him playing, 'This Year's Love', on the piano in the drawing room, although of course I didn't know the song was going to be such a huge hit. I found David to be a quiet, gentle person, who was always thoughtful and considered in everything he said. He seemed very at home in the Park, and we did our best to make sure he was given the space he needed to write and rehearse. It was fascinating to see his process, how the songs evolved during the two weeks he was with us.

I also got to meet Bryan Ferry, the hero of my youth. Years later, I discovered that he wrote part of the *Avalon* album while staying in the West of Ireland, and several of his band members, particularly Andy Mackay, have come to stay with us. Andy and I have become great friends over the years, and he has been kind enough to introduce me to the iconic singer, and allow me to spend time in the studio with the band. Andy is massively talented, a multi-instrumentalist and a genuinely nice guy who also loves restaurants and good food, and this is one of the reasons we get on so well. His classical training brought much of the innovation to the heyday of Roxy Music and its ever-changing tone during the band's career. Each of their eight studio albums is different, enthralling and exquisitely produced. But then, so is Andy's band leader.

I've been in the studio with Bryan, and while of course I love watching him perform, and being close up when he delivers a vocal is an incredible experience, what really interested me was watching the sound engineers at work: observing how someone could alter the sound by turning a dial, moving a fader, directing an instrument from one speaker to another was an eye-opener. At one point, I watched as an amplifier was moved from one side of the studio to another, to better bounce that guitar sound off a particular wall, to create resonance. That kind of attention to detail is something I understand very well. And seeing how records are produced, the craft that goes into them, just made me appreciate music all the more.

I recently came across an interview with Dallas Schoo, the sound technician for U2's The Edge. Dallas has worked with him for 33 years, and a huge part of what he does involves preparing the guitars. That means he knows what particular strings are used on each different model – D'Adarrio on the Gibson Les Paul, Ernie Bell on the Fender and so on. He understands that for the song 'Bad', the guitar Edge uses needs to be tuned down a semi-tone to match the sampled keyboards they use, and that adding a tiny amount of reverb will alter the pitch perfectly. Dallas knows the specifics of the 26 guitars The Edge plays in each concert, and he also knows the needs of these instruments will be different if they are taken into a studio.

The music on a record alone does not communicate the anguish, skill and sweat that went into making it. The years of experience behind the craft. You do not become U2, Bruce Springsteen or The Rolling Stones without decades of hard graft and a laser-like attention to detail.

And then there's the lifestyle of the musician. I can identify with it a little bit, and most people have no idea how difficult it can be. Dan Fogelberg has a lovely lyric in his song 'Same Old Lang Syne'. In the song he bumps into his ex-girlfriend and she says she came across one of his albums in a record store, and assumes he must be doing very well. In this song, he makes a wistful response about the audience being heavenly but the travelling hell – a line I came to respect a few years later. People who have never had to travel constantly for work attach great glamour to the touring life. London, New York, LA, Hong Kong, Sydney … they seem all very glamorous and exciting but the reality is quite different. Suitcase living is horrible no matter where you are.

Music taught me that creating something beautiful can sometimes carry a heavy cost on the innovator. And sometimes, you just have to be prepared to pay it.

Beezies and Me

During the school holidays and at weekends I worked for Damien in Beezies. Starting in washing up, where I had to stand on a box to reach the sink, I got my first taste of a busy kitchen when I was 11. It was hard work, but I came to love the buzz of conversation, the orders being shouted out, the hiss of steam and the clatter of pots. There were other things I liked less: the greasy water I spent hours up to my elbows in, and the smell of so many different meals all being cooked at the same time that you could never get out of your clothes.

Beezies did over 300 covers a night, so the plates and cups and knives and forks just kept coming. It was high pressure, there was no time to dawdle and if it was really busy, you didn't get any break. But the camaraderie was amazing, and even though I was so young, once the kitchen crew saw I could hold my own, I was welcomed into their pirate crew with open arms. It was a special feeling.

As time passed and I grew a few inches I progressed to the floor to collecting glasses. It was my first encounter with the public and I loved it, too. The clientele at Beezies was varied and never less than interesting. I've always been a people watcher, and my brother's bar gave me ample opportunity. Business people, politicians, musicians, actors, artists, writers, alcoholics, families, off-duty Gardaí, doctors, butchers, travelling salesmen, farmers, builders, land developers, depressives, wannabe comedians, teachers, priests, gangsters, chancers, geniuses and fools – I dealt with them all, and it was without doubt the best training ground I could have found.

By the time I was 14, I could have a conversation with someone from any walk of life without feeling intimidated or belittled. This was a significant change from the kid who felt so out of place walking in the gates of CUS, but in the environment of the busy pub, it just felt as if the playing field was more level. Working on the floor, front of house, I soon understood that people came in looking to find a connection. They wanted you to be their friend. So striking up a rapport was automatically easier, less strained. It was like pushing an open door.

The pub honed my instincts, too. You had to know when someone wanted to talk, and when they wanted to be left alone. When they needed a listening ear, and when they wanted to lead the conversation. When they wanted you to laugh at their jokes and when they needed to sob on your shoulder.

Beezies was formative for another reason, too. Working with Damien taught me that every single person in a pub, restaurant or hotel is important. Everyone has a role to play, and if one person isn't pulling their weight, it impacts on everyone else.

I was just a kid who washed up and collected glasses, but if I was too slow, or my work was second-rate, it meant someone else would have to stop doing what they were doing to help me out, and that meant their station was affected. You needed to be prepared to do anything, too – if the kitchen was slammed I was pulled back there from the floor to peel spuds or wash up again. If the sink was blocked, I would be handed a plunger. When someone got sick in the toilets, I was there with a mop and bucket. And there was no point in complaining, because Damian would have been doing it himself if he had the time. It was just the way working in a busy establishment like that was.

Despite my young age and relative inexperience, I was never treated with anything other than the height of respect, and when the staff were winding down after a hard night, I was included (although I was given a glass of Coke as opposed to the pints they consumed). To get everyone out at closing time you had to pull the fuse on the juke box and turn on all the lights fully. Then, when they were all gone, we would turn the juke box back on and have an hour of music at the expense of the customers who never got to hear the song they paid for. As a result, I can tell you every note of Gary Numan's 'Cars', with its staccato drums and wonderful electronic bass line. Because of this sense of inclusion, I would have done anything for any of the guys and girls who worked alongside me, and I knew instinctively they would do the same for me.

Damien sold the pub to open a restaurant in Rosses Point called Reveries. I never worked there as by then I had moved on. But I will always remember my time in that amazing pub as one of the most important and significant in my life. The skills I learned there I continue to use to this day.

CIDER AND MATHS

I left Beezies to work at Bourke's Fruit and Veg wholesalers, becoming part of a team that worked a truck that supplied hotels, shops and supermarkets along a route from Sligo to Ballina. The job involved early starts and being on the road for long hours, but it showed me a completely different side of the business, which I found just as fascinating as the one I'd seen in Beezies.

I learned there are lots of little tricks of the trade. For example, shopkeepers always checked the top tray of apples and oranges to test the quality of the produce. But never the second tray. From my time on that truck, I know to always check the second tray, as nine out of every ten will have either a missing apple or a rotten one. My suppliers now know not to try and foist sub-standard fruit and veg on me. I'm wise to them.

While I was learning the ropes with Bourke's, I was continuing my studies in Ballisodare. I was having lots of fun, but I was beginning to understand in a practical sense that Harvard or Yale were never going to feature in my future. So when the Intermediate Certificate (now the Junior Certificate) loomed on the horizon, I was already looking at options. I knew I needed to start building towards a future that would be meaningful to me, and I had to find a way to get there that suited my talents and abilities.

So while I was committed to doing the Inter Cert, if I'm honest, I didn't approach it with the weighty seriousness I'd been told these exams merited. And I found the experience of sitting them intolerably boring. I found it so pointless to be sitting in a long exam hall, surrounded by other students, their heads all bowed, scratching away at their sheets of paper, answering questions and solving problems I felt offered nothing to me or the life I wanted to lead.

In those days you weren't allowed to leave an exam until the last hour, and most of the exams were at least two hours, some longer, and I felt trapped and irritable. On the morning of the Maths paper my mates Bosco, Conor and I 'borrowed' three bikes from the school yard and went to O'Callaghan's Pub in Ballygawley, where we persuaded the publican to sell us three flagons of cider, which we drank in a convenient field we found on the return trip. It was a beautiful, sunny morning, and the ice-cold cider seemed the perfect accompaniment to the gorgeous summer weather. The three of us lay off in the long grass, listening to the Meadow Larks and the Pipits, and the worry of having to sit a standardised Maths test just drifted away. For a few hours, anyway.

With the determination only a certain degree of drunkenness can bestow on a man, we hauled ourselves upright with very little time to spare, and (I'm ashamed to admit) wobbily piloted our purloined bicycles back to the exam hall, where the invigilator studiously ignored the fact we were reeking of alcohol and were virtually cross-eyed from drink. In a sure sign that God protects the confused and infirm, I got an A in that Maths exam, although I have little memory of completing it.

On the Friday of that first week of the Inter Cert, having sat five of my nine scheduled exams I knew I'd had enough, and I informed my mother I would not be returning to school on Monday to finish my state exams. She must have been horrified, but she took the news with calm acceptance, and informed me that, as long as I had a job to go to, she would give me her blessing.

I made a phone call, and ten minutes after making my decision, I had a full-time job on Bourke's Vegetable Truck. I was about to embark upon the world of work. My real adventures were about to begin.

Finding a Different Path

I started full time on the vegetable truck the following Monday and, much to my mother and father's credit, they never berated me or questioned my life choice. As a parent, I now understand this was either an expression of total confidence, or that maybe they were just keeping their powder dry while they waited for me to fall flat on my face. Luckily, I kept my footing – for the first few months, at least.

There were other kids in my class who did not have the supportive home base I did, and I watched quite a few of them head off to third-level courses they were absolutely unsuited for, meaning more than a few of them either dropped out or wasted three years of their lives studying something they were destined never to achieve employment in.

We live in a world where mental health problems are at epidemic levels. I have come to believe a huge proportion of these very serious and debilitating emotional conditions are caused by the stress young people experience due to the peer pressure to be something they are not. How many kids who might be best suited to manual work, or to serving in a bar, or cooking, or farming, end up being pushed into doing degrees they neither want nor need, because that is what society dictates they must do?

I have employed many young people over the years and I would say about half of them are suitable for third-level academia. The other half excel in service roles, trades or in sales. The accepted wisdom, though, is that jobs like that are somehow 'less' – that they don't deliver the same sense of achievement or satisfaction. Well I'm here to tell you, that really is not the case.

From the moment I made the decision not to return to that exam hall, I have gone to bed every evening knowing I made the correct decision, and I have lived a full, exciting and successful life. I work alongside people I admire and respect, and the majority have never set foot inside the hallowed halls of a university. Yet they are none the worse for it. And here's another side of the argument you might not have considered – universities and colleges are in fact businesses. They need enrolment to maintain the registration fees and grants that keep them open. The courses they offer are also getting longer and longer to keep students in the system. Think about it.

When I left school, you could go to college to get a national certificate, which could be achieved in two years and would qualify you for many jobs. There were also diplomas, which took three years, and degrees generally took four. People who had achieved Bachelor of Arts degrees were seen as highly qualified individuals indeed.

Not anymore. Today's school leaver is expected to acquire either a Master's or a PhD before they will even be considered for an interview for many positions. Just think about that for a moment. Children spend eight years in primary school; six years in secondary; four years as an under-graduate; and as many as five as a post-grad. That's 23 years in education, with no guarantee of a job at the end of it. And if they are not naturally academic, society is sentencing these kids to a veritable prison sentence of unhappiness.

So basically, the country has potentially paid for 23 years of education for someone with a post-graduate qualification. That person works for perhaps 40 years, followed by a pension for another 20 years or thereabouts. What this means is that the State has paid for 43 years, or about half of that person's time on the planet. I haven't had a flagon of cider today, but that piece of arithmetic seems odd to say the least, and I don't know how sustainable it is.

Many of these youngsters would be so much happier if they were given some guidance and support to help them find an alternative pathway to what they really want to do. We need to see the value in simpler, more instinctive labour. Because the world can't function without plasterers and waiters and painter-decorators and chefs. I am always struck when I encounter middle-aged waiters in other countries and admire how they dedicated their lives to service, not feeling any stigma about performing this level of job at an older age. I always make a point of tipping them well. They keep the show on the road and deserve the reward. As do sixteen-year-olds who work on vegetable trucks.

A Minor Misstep

Thankfully my mother and father did not bow to such societal pressures, and I took off at 7 a.m. on Monday morning in the Bourke's Hino truck. The days were busy, the work simple loading and unloading.

What I loved about it though, was that four days a week we got lunch in whichever restaurants were convenient to wherever we dropped off at midday. I looked forward to these lunches immensely – the food could be hit and miss, but I thoroughly enjoyed soaking in the ambience and seeing how the various places ran their service.

Having worked in Beezies, I had a sense of how things should be done. I knew what made a restaurant tick, and I could tell right off if somewhere was well run or if the chef or manager didn't have their eye on the ball. I didn't realise it then, but those lunchbreaks were a learning experience.

On Wednesdays we delivered to Belmullet, in County Mayo, and had to bring sandwiches for lunch as no restaurant was open outside the summer months. I must have been completely spoiled at that point, because I found these lunchtimes unbearably grim. We ate in the truck overlooking an idyllic beach with an apple, orange or plum – taken from the second tray, of course.

I enjoyed working on the truck, but I knew it wasn't forever, and after a month I began looking for something better, and thought I found it in Musgraves Cash and Carry.

I was wrong; it was my first real misstep, and it just about gave my long-suffering mother a hernia.

I didn't mind the work, which wasn't hugely unlike what I'd done on the truck: it was primarily unloading pallets and stacking their contents on shelves; or the reverse, helping customers fill their orders and carrying stuff out to their trucks or vans.

The problem I had was the ethos of the place. Everywhere else I worked there was a buzz, a sense of fun or creativity and a desire to do the best job you could do. Not here. It was boring, regimented and joyless. No one seemed interested in what they were doing, and in the brief time I was there, I saw people doing the most half-hearted work I have ever seen. The supervisors didn't even seem to care. I lasted a day. I must have shown some promise, because the manager came to see Mum and Dad to try and talk me back, but there was no way I would even hear of it.

I cannot imagine how my parents must have felt. I had left school on the understanding I was doing so to go to a full-time job. And here I was, turning my nose up at a well-paid one where the boss actually came to my home, begging me to go back. But once again, they placed their trust in me that I knew what I was doing; which was just as well. I was about to make my final career leap into the hotel business. And once I made that jump, I never looked back.

The Ballroom of No Romance

That Christmas, Jim Feeney, the General Manager of the Sligo Park Hotel, gave me a job in the bar. The Sligo Park held a soft spot in my heart for several reasons. Both Damien and Francis had worked there, and it had the dubious honour of being where I attended my first disco. Which is a story in itself.

In those days there were 'teenage discos' held during mid-term breaks and school holidays. They were the cause of great excitement, and some pals and I decided to go along one night to the Sligo Park to see what it was all about.

I must have been 13 or 14, and an outing such as this was very much a rite of passage, or so I thought. The place was packed with crowds of boys and girls standing around in groups looking at each other, everyone seemingly afraid to cross the Rubicon and actually strike up a conversation, never mind ask for a dance.

It was dark, extremely noisy and, this being two decades before the Irish government outlawed smoking in public spaces, the dance hall was shrouded in a fog of tobacco smoke, making it almost impossible to either see or hear the person you were supposed to be asking onto the floor for a dance, and (hopefully) a shift.

As the night progressed, myself and my friend, James, decided it was time to make a move. We determined we would ask two girls we had identified on the other side of the floor, which I had started to think of as 'enemy territory'.

'I'll ask the one on the left, you go for the one on the right,' I bellowed at James over the thumping music.

He shouted something back which I took as agreement (I couldn't hear a thing), and we took deep breaths of smoky air, and broke cover, making a beeline for our prospective dance partners.

With shouted words and a few hand signals, we got the girls to understand what we were proposing, and I got what I can only describe as a half-commitment to dance. I couldn't work out what was wrong – I thought I was being very smooth, but it seemed the young lady I was attempting to chat up was very unwilling to part company with her girlfriend.

I cast an eye over at James, and saw he was in deep conversation with her friend.

'He seems to be getting on way better than me,' I thought ruefully.

I figured I'd better up my game, and complimented her on her hair, her outfit, her makeup ... nothing seemed to be working. In fact, she just appeared to be getting more and more uncomfortable. Finally, I looked over, and saw James was gone. I caught a glimpse of him disappearing out the rear entrance to the hall and decided I would give it up as a bad job. Wishing the clearly disinterested young lady a good night, I followed my friend, who was leaning against the wall outside looking very sheepish indeed.

'What happened?' I demanded to know. 'You looked like you were well in there!'

'I definitely wasn't,' he said. 'Not even close.'

'Me neither,' I said. 'I used every line I could think of, but she wasn't leaving her friend. I don't think she was into me.'

'Oh, I used every line too,' James admitted. 'But I ran into one major problem.'

'I'm listening.'

'The "girl" I was trying to get on the dance floor wasn't a girl at all. It was the boyfriend of the girl you were talking to. He just happens to have long hair and a taste for silk shirts.'

James and I gazed at each other for a moment before bursting into laughter. We walked home, gutted our night had been such a dead loss in the romance stakes.

JOHN BRENNAN, CHEF

I worked in the bar at the Sligo Park that Christmas, and I loved it. It felt good to be back working with people, and I understood how to put customers at ease. Christmas was a busy time at the hotel, too, and I thrived in the hustle and bustle of the place.

My experience in the cash and carry, however, as well as those memories of La Touche, not to mention the fun I'd had in the kitchen in Beezies, had got me thinking. Maybe the kitchen was where my heart truly lay. Would it be possible for me to recreate those fantastic chips, to be behind someone else's cherished taste memories?

I decided I'd like to try my hand at it, and that January I started a chef's course in Clonskeagh in Dublin. The awarding body was CERT, the Community Education Response Training body, and this Introductory Cookery Course ran for thirteen weeks. It covered all the basics and offered a great insight into kitchen management and operations. I really enjoyed it. The building where we worked is now the large mosque in Clonskeagh, and I stayed with my sister Catherine in Ballinteer, which wasn't far away. There were 12 of us in my class group, and we were all set up in pairs at workstations spaced out around the large training room. Each station had a hob, a chopping board, knives and utensils, and the one opposite was its exact mirror image.

We learned knife skills; the basics of butchering meat; culinary hygiene; economy of movement; the hierarchy of a professional kitchen. We were taught how to make a stock from scratch and how to dress a plate. The course showed us everything you need to know to work in a kitchen. I knew most of it already from my time at Beezies, so I was one of the star pupils. It was the first time in my life I'd been top of the class, and it was a fantastic feeling.

An important part of the course was to complete several sessions of on-the-job training, where we were sent out to work in actual kitchens, usually to bolster the existing staff when they had a large function. One of mine was at a large hotel in Dublin (I won't name it, for obvious reasons). The occasion was a huge dinner dance at which a significant number of dignitaries and celebrities were present, and the tension in the kitchen was palpable. This was, in many ways, a showcase for the chef and the events team.

As a student I was placed on starters, and my job was to plate them up: I had a bowl full of washed salad leaves and squeeze bottles of dressing and sauce. The sous-chef would pass me pieces of grilled trout, which I had to stick on the plate, dress, and garnish with a selection of leaves. Not rocket science, but when you have to do 200 of them quickly, you need to have your wits about you.

It became obvious to me by the third or fourth plate that something was wrong. The pieces of trout that were coming to my station were not cooked at all, and some were still frozen. I knew that if something like this were to happen in Beezies, Damien would go mad. I thought about that, and decided I'd better do something about it. I was only a student, after all, and wasn't getting paid. They couldn't exactly fire me.

I approached the Head Chef, a giant of a man in a starched white jacket, his face bright red and wreathed in sweat.

'I'm sorry Chef, but the trout I'm getting is still raw.'

He glowered at me.

'Show me.'

I brought him to the few plates I'd done, and showed him the selection of other pieces, each one worse than the one that went before it.

'What would you do if you were me?' he asked.

'It's too late to fix the trout,' I said. 'If you have some smoked salmon in the storeroom, I can use that. No one will know it's not smoked trout if I dress it right. It's not ideal, but it'll do in a pinch.'

He smiled at me, squeezed my shoulder, and that is exactly what we did.

I had three job offers by the time I graduated, and needless to say, my mother was over the moon. And I was quite pleased with myself, too. I accepted a position in The Abbot in Monkstown and was due to start the following Monday. I travelled home that weekend, planning on relaxing before starting a job I knew would consume most of my waking hours for the foreseeable future. And that may have been my second misstep.

While home I slipped on the pond across the road from my parents' house, which, covered in thick ice, my mates and I were using for a spot of impromptu skating. It was quite a tumble, and I broke my collar bone, putting me on the flat of my back and out of action for three months. Needless to say, I lost the job, and in 1982 there were not many jobs to be had.

It was another brief moment of despair, but to his eternal credit Mr Feeney gave me my old job back in the bar of the Sligo Park Hotel. And so began 13 great years in that wonderful workplace.

PART THREE

Climbing the Ladder

The Domino Effect of One Decision

The Sligo Park Hotel was a commercial hotel owned by an Irish family, who were also involved in the Jurys chain. It was professional and comfortable without stepping over into the realm of luxury. The hotel was the business hub for the region, hosting board meetings, national conferences and trade fairs, but locals saw it as part of their community and never failed to use the services too, having family meals in the restaurant, celebrating christenings, first communions and confirmations. Meanwhile the bar had many regulars who only ever came in for pints and never utilised any of the hotel's other services at all.

So working in the bar forced me to make use of the interpersonal skills I'd developed at Beezies to maximum effect. I saw every walk of life come in and out those bar doors, and I was expected to engage with them all and make them feel valued and welcome, whether that person was an elderly farmer in for his couple of pints of Guinness, or an executive staying over on his way to Belfast.

At the Sligo Park I also, for the first time, saw how badly thought-out management decisions, particularly around the very important area of costing, could have widespread detrimental effects.

Mr Feeney left to pursue a job elsewhere, and a new general manager came to us from Limerick. I don't know precisely what his management credentials were, but whatever they were, past experience had clearly not prepared him for the challenge of running a commercial hotel in a small Irish town. In the first month of his appointment, our new captain made the decision to raise the banqueting price from £12.50 to £16. This meant that if a company was holding a conference with us and, as was the norm for such occasions, wanted to put on a dinner for all the attendees, they had to pay £16 per head for each meal, a hike of £3.50. Which, if there were 100 people in attendance, added a cost of £350. Back in 1982 that was an awful lot of money.

The folly of such an enormous jump was pointed out to him by everyone, but he was absolutely adamant, claiming the hotel was undercutting itself and that nowhere in the country was there a banqueting rate so ridiculously low as £12.50. That may have been the case, but it seems no one told our clients the news. In quick succession we lost the Rotary Annual Gala, then the Chamber of Commerce Dinner. In a slow and painful drip, event after event that had been hosted by our hotel for years took its business elsewhere. It was an unmitigated disaster and the following year proved very quiet as a result, resulting in an impact that was much more than just fiscal.

Staff morale became extremely low, and when morale is low, the standard of work suffers. People stop taking pride in their jobs, things are done in a slipshod manner and mistakes get made. The department heads within the hotel had to work extra hard to bring their teams into line, and in the end everyone pulled together to get the ship back on an even keel.

As a result of losing so many prestigious events, the hotel was no longer routinely mentioned in the local papers. That's another thing people tend not to think about – if you happen to be hosting the Chamber of Commerce Dinner in your dining room, the photographer from the newspaper comes along to take photos of all the local dignitaries, and when those photos appear in the supplement in the paper, the caption will read: *Mr and Mrs Jones, enjoying their evening at the Chamber of Commerce Christmas Party at the Sligo Park Hotel.* This is free advertising, and the hotel lost almost all of it when the events and functions went elsewhere.

I don't want to labour the point, but that type of advertising is something you just can't buy. It keeps the hotel in the minds and consciousness of the local community the whole year around, and when a family is thinking about where to have their daughter's wedding or where they'll take the mourners after a funeral, the hotel will be the first place that pops into their heads, because the name is so familiar.

The Sligo Park experienced a couple of very lean years because of that single costing decision. I can only imagine the discussions and debates that were had during meetings with the family who owned the hotel and the other stakeholders, but the manager stalwartly stood his ground, insisting he was playing a long game.

I have no idea whether or not he was being truthful and if the tough times we worked through were part of a grand scheme only he understood, but I must finish the story by admitting the business, slowly but surely, did return at the higher price point. It seems that the excellent level of service the hotel always maintained, as well as the overall quality of the experience, won out over price. At any rate, we were back in business and it was a good lesson. Service and quality deserve a premium price. Value cannot only be judged by cost; other places might have been cheaper but they were not as good value, hence the clients all came back. The manager was right, though it took us a long time to see it.

A Brennan Brother Walks Into a Bar ...
and Builds Some Contacts

S tationed in the bar at the Sligo Park, I was ideally situated to meet all kinds of influential people, and I used that vantage point to build a network of contacts I still use today.

The medical industry was on a roll in the early 1980s – it always performs well during a recession – and reps from lots of different companies stayed with us weekly, so we got to know them very well. One day one of them, Maurice Kennedy, who worked for a company called Medical Services Limited, confided in me over a drink that his company could not source wooden products like side tables, wobble boards and bed trays.

I enquired as to where someone might learn the dimensions and material specifications for such items, and he told me he could get me a booklet outlining what was required. To my delight, the following week Maurice handed me a supplier's catalogue that told me exactly what hospitals, health centres and rehabilitation centres expected in their wooden equipment – the sizes, thicknesses, safety parameters all carefully laid out.

Of course, this wasn't much good to me – I could knock up a mean Christmas log, but sculpting a bed tray or constructing a rolling table was more than a little beyond my skillset. However, I did know someone who could help. I contacted a school friend, Bosco Kearins, who was the most talented woodworker I'd met at my time in Ballisodare – the one who could handle a flagon of cider before a Maths exam. He could build almost anything, and when we sat down to look at the specs, I saw his face light up. I knew I'd found the right partner.

We built some prototypes, wrote a business plan and made an application to the Industrial Development Authority. It seemed a long shot, and I wasn't pinning my hopes on it. Ireland was in the throes of a deep recession in the early eighties and we were two 18-year-old kids with absolutely no experience whatsoever in the field of constructing and selling medical equipment.

We must have made a good pitch though, because we were awarded a grant of £87,000, which, by any definition, was a lot of money back in 1983. With all the brashness of youth we proceeded to open a factory in Sligo Town. It was an extremely exciting time, and I revelled in making it all happen.

I already had a good venue in mind, a storage building on the northern edge of Sligo Town that had been lying idle for about a year. I negotiated a lease with the owner that was very competitive, and now we had a base of operations.

Bosco had a few friends who were great carpenters, and they had friends in the trade too, and within the space of a couple of days we had a team of skilled craftsworkers to make our product. Between us, we had no difficulty sourcing wood and tools, and we were off to a flying start. It was as if all the lessons I'd learned from my father and from Damien and from watching and listening and learning in the Sligo

Park were all put into action. Four months almost to the day after we received our grant I filled the van with samples of our various products and hit the road for Dublin for my first sales trip.

I'm not going to bore you with the details. Suffice it to say that I returned two days later with half those goods still on board. We had, quite simply, miscalculated and made too many of some items and not enough of others. In short, we hadn't researched the market thoroughly enough – we'd been arrogant and were now left with stock, a physical reminder of profits we did not have but which carried a cost. It was an expensive lesson and one I never forgot: don't make what you haven't sold and make sure what you do make is as good as it can possibly be.

Understanding we had bitten off more than we could chew with the field of medical supplies, we altered our focus and made bespoke kitchens, dining room tables, cupboards and work desks for anyone who approached us and was prepared to pay what we asked. By changing our focus, we jumped from a niche client group to the mainstream, and that is a place I never like to be. It offers few challenges and can easily staunch creativity. As soon as that shift occurred, I knew my time in the furniture business was going to be short lived.

Add to that the fact that I was working 80 hours a week between the hotel and the factory, trying to give my all to both projects, and you had a recipe that could never work. As it happened, the universe stepped in and took the choice away from me in the end.

We used Iroko wood, which is a beautiful material but generates a huge amount of choking dust. During my adventure in the world of furniture making, I learned that I have inherited my father's chest, and breathing in great clouds of teak dust was not benefitting me at all. So it was that after two years of producing some pretty fine wood-crafted furniture we closed up shop, me to continue my journey into the world of hotels, and Bosco to become one of the biggest manufacturers of stairs in the country. It had been a steep learning curve for both of us, but the lessons we learned were not wasted.

Feck the Begrudgers

Shortly after opening the factory, I ran into the woodwork teacher from Ballisodare as I was heading into work in the Sligo Park. I had never distinguished myself in his class, and I had a sneaking suspicion he did not harbour many warm feelings towards me.

'Well Brennan,' he said, and I knew from the tone of his voice that he had a chip the size of a two by four on his shoulder, 'I hear you opened a woodworking factory.'

'I did,' I retorted, and I gave him one of the grins I used on drunk customers who had just told me the same joke for the millionth time and stuffed up the punchline to boot.

I knew this man was bitter about my apparent success, and it annoyed me, because I was putting in a superhuman effort, working every hour God sent and not exactly earning a huge amount for all my blood, sweat and tears. I wasn't going to give him the satisfaction of showing him I was at the end of my rope.

'Well, Brennan,' my former teacher said through clenched teeth. 'I can tell you right here and now you couldn't join your hands never mind two pieces of timber.'

I laughed out loud at that.

'You might be right,' I replied, 'but I did get a savage grant from the IDA, and you never had the balls to do anything worthwhile for yourself.'

I saw all the colour drain from his face at that.

'So better to try and fail than never to try at all,' I finished.

I was bone tired, but I went into work that day with a smile on my face.

Saying Goodbye to Dad

We lost Dad on 29 February 1988, while I was working between the Sligo Park and the furniture factory. It was sad, and we were all heartbroken, but it was also an end to his suffering. He'd had as good a life as he could while still being compromised, and in those final days we took turns being with him when he was too weak to get around.

I was working in the factory the morning he died, and a family friend called in to say I should ring home. I ran to the nearest phone box and was told by my sister Susan that Dad had died. I remember standing there on the quiet street, wondering how I was supposed to feel.

Losing a parent is a monumental thing, and my dad, sick and all as he was, had always been such a huge presence, and an unorthodox man in many ways, yet steady, reliable and stable. A good role model, a loving parent and an inspiration. I decided there and then all I could do was honour him by being the best version of myself I could be. And I've tried to stick to that since that day.

Dad continued his unique way of approaching life even in death. He left his body to medical science, which meant we didn't have a funeral in the immediate wake of his death. We had a Mass to mark his passing, and then his remains were taken to Galway, where they could be used to help medical science better understand the impact of emphysema on the lungs and the circulatory system. He was returned to us two years later, and we had the funeral then. It wasn't the usual course of events for saying goodbye to a loved one, but then, I don't like the usual. I'd far rather do things a little differently. I got that from my dad.

Discos in the Hills of Donegal

I continued to work in the Sligo Park, but that didn't stop me from capitalising on other opportunities when they presented themselves. I really do believe that the key to success is recognising an opportunity when you see it, and grabbing on with both hands so it doesn't scoot on by.

My cousin, who also carries the illustrious name of John Brennan and is now a noted Maths teacher (I'm told he manages without the cider), had the agency for glow sticks which he sold at concerts in Dublin. A glow stick is a self-contained plastic tube that contains chemicals which, when combined, become luminescent – basically, they glow. Once the light is activated (you do this by bending the tube, which breaks a seal inside, causing the elements to mix) it can't be switched off, and it will give light for a couple of hours before dimming and going out.

These natty little objects were designed for use by the military during night manoeuvres, but the fact they came in a variety of bright, fluorescent colours (pinks, blues and greens) made them hugely popular on the nightclub and party circuit, and that's where my similarly monikered cousin sold them. On a visit one weekend, I went along with him as he hopped from one Dublin hotspot to another, and to my amazement I saw he couldn't sell the things fast enough. People were falling over themselves to buy them.

I remember standing by the wall of Lillie's Bordello, a famous Dublin venue, seeing the entire place lit up by my cousin's glow sticks: a sea of pink and blue tubes bobbing up and down in time to the music. Looking around the club, it occurred to me that the sticks themselves told you where to go in the nightclub to sell them. From my vantage point, I could see an area that was unilluminated. I pointed it out to John, and five minutes later it too was glowing pink. And the money rolled in.

I had to get in on this opportunity. At that time the nightclub business was massive, and the North West had a growing number of huge venues, many of them in far-flung and isolated places to avoid noise complaints. Vast convoys of buses shipped people in from all over the region. Some of these places would comfortably bring in 3000 people on a Saturday night. I knew that if I could bring glow sticks to the North, I'd be on to a winner.

Donegal was a Mecca for clubbers. They came from far and wide to dance the night away in a couple of famous nightspots: The Holly Rood (which I immediately thought was a good omen) which was located near Bundoran, and The Limelight, just outside Glenties. The Limelight was the one I really wanted to infiltrate, as the word on the street was that on a good night 5000 people packed its dance floors. So off I went one Sunday afternoon to see if I couldn't ingratiate myself with the owner.

I was in luck when I arrived at the sprawling building from which The Limelight operated, as the young man who ran the club was there stocking the bar. I liked that, as it reminded me of myself – here was a man who was in charge of one of the biggest nightclubs in the country, but he wasn't afraid to do the menial jobs. I knew we'd get on. When I told him why I was there he asked for £100 up front as a kind of trading licence. This I knew from my cousin was a standard arrangement, and I agreed immediately.

'If you really want to see if your glow sticks will sell here, you're going to want to be here on Hallowe'en night,' the young owner informed me as I was leaving. 'It's one of the busiest nights of the year.'

'How busy?' I asked.

'Seven thousand people will pass through those doors that night,' he laughed. 'That busy enough for you?'

Now all I had to do was make sure I wasn't rostered to work in the Sligo Park that night! As luck would have it, I wasn't, and I ordered 7000 sticks in the most popular colours from John, then commandeered two friends to come with me.

I had, by now, started seeing a pretty young girl who worked in an insurance firm in Sligo. Her name was Gwen, and she and I seemed to make a good team, so I asked her to come along as well. I was driving a Ford Fiesta van in those days, so with the two lads stretched out in the back, we headed for the hills of Donegal.

There were 27 buses parked outside at eight o'clock, even though the club didn't open its doors until 10. We knew right away the owner hadn't been exaggerating.

'Get your selling faces on,' I told my little team. 'This is going to be a crazy night.'

I wasn't wrong. We waited until 11 before going in, by which time there must have been over 50 buses outside and too many cars to count. Our stock was made up of 4000 yellow sticks, 2000 red sticks and 1000 blue ones, which reflected the popularity of each colour, according to the few nights I'd spent selling them with my cousin.

'Let's go with the yellow first and see how we go,' I told my fellow salespeople.

The Limelight was in fact three nightclubs in one: two discos, each pumping out a different style of music, and one bar with a live band on a good-sized stage. Gwen stayed by the door, and each of us boys took a room and off we went. With so many people and no such thing as mobile phones we decided to all take 200 sticks and meet back at the car in half an hour to compare notes. Gwen could keep track of our movements, as the yellow sticks appeared like beacons as we moved around the rooms.

We didn't have to wait 30 minutes. In fact, we were all back at the car in 10. I bought the glow sticks for 50p each, and we sold them for £1. And in 10 minutes, we had just sold 600 sticks and had £600. This was wonderful, but it presented us with a problem we had not foreseen. We had too much money to mind and nowhere secure to keep it. The disco-goers were so delighted with our product, people actually left the club to follow us out to the car park in search of more!

Gwen offered to stay in the van to look after the money, and my two intrepid pals and I returned with the remaining yellow sticks and within another 10 minutes were sold out. We now had a cool £4000 in cash on our persons.

I was slightly overwhelmed, and the two boys were incredulous – they'd never seen anything like it. I needed to breathe and think, so we went out to the van and took it up the road a short distance.

'This is amazing,' Gwen kept saying. 'I've never seen so much money in one bundle before!'

Neither had I. It was exhilarating, but strange.

After an hour we went back and this time parked in a different area of the car park – I was so aware that all this loose cash could draw a lot of unwanted attention from the wrong type of person, and I was suddenly mindful of the safety of my friends. And Gwen even more so. As we only had 2000 red sticks, and given what had just happened that meant they would be a hot property, we decided to up our price to the princely sum of £2.

'Right lads, take a deep breath and let's do this,' I said, and in we went.

We were swamped. Within 15 minutes the sticks were gone and people were climbing over one another to get to us. We now had £8000 and the glove compartment of the van couldn't hold any more. I took up the floor in the back and stuffed as much as possible around the spare wheel.

That left us with the blue sticks. The crowd was waiting for us at the door, and three minutes later we were on the road to Sligo with £10,000 in small bills. It was an incredible night; one I will never forget.

I learned an unforgettable lesson in the power of market demand, and how important it is to manage your stock and time your sales. Never again would I make the mistakes I had made with the hospital furniture. It felt as if I had vindicated myself.

And Gwen and I went to the Canaries for two weeks on the proceeds. It was a perfect way to celebrate. We had a fantastic holiday (I don't think I've ever gotten a better suntan!) and we shared our apartment complex with some lovely people. It's funny, because while I've never set eyes on them again, I remember them really well – there was one couple from Adamstown in Wexford, for example.

I returned from the Canaries with my batteries recharged, ready for the next adventure.

The Leisure Business and Beyond

The effort and energy I put into my work at the bar in the Sligo Park was noticed and I was promoted to Sales Manager, a job that came with an office – the first one I'd had in my career and, now that I think about it, the only one. It wasn't a big office; it didn't have a window overlooking anything very pretty, but it was an acknowledgment of the hard work I'd been doing, and I was very proud of it.

The hotel was just about to open a new leisure centre, and it was seen as an opportunity to rebrand and relaunch the business. We were moving from a regional hotel to something a bit more upmarket, a bit more cutting edge, and management wanted to inject the staff with a new lease of life, and let our regulars know we were developing something special that would benefit them, too.

Leisure centres were a very new thing at the time, so as the newly appointed Sales Manager I was sent off to visit the Newport Hotel in Kilkenny, the Limerick Inn and Jurys in Cork to take a look at their recently opened leisure facilities and see what I could learn. It was a wonderful opportunity, as I got to see the operating procedures in all of these locations. The hotels I was sent to were much bigger than the Sligo Park and all based in parts of the country with much more competition. The management teams were sharper, hungrier and completely focused on the daily battle they had to engage in for every scrap of business.

I was inspired by them. They made me see how easy it is to become complacent, and how that complacency can make you dull and lethargic if you let it. The lesson I took from my tour of these amazing hotels was that every single customer, no matter how small the interaction, should be seen as a victory. An achievement.

Something as mundane as giving a guest directions to the theatre where they are seeing a show is an opportunity to promote your hotel and earn that guest's loyalty. Making sure the sinks are spotless in the bathrooms at your leisure centre sends a message to your clients that you care about their welfare. Making sure each and every one of your bar staff know how to pull the perfect pint of Guinness every time they step up to the tap builds a reputation for excellence that will, by association, cross over into other aspects of your operation. On my research trip, I made sure I soaked up all the wisdom I could, and returned to Sligo determined to use every last scrap of it.

Political Activism

Opening a leisure centre proved to be much more labour intensive than I had ever imagined. What should the membership fees be? I knew what they charged in Kilkenny and I knew what they asked for in Cork, but Sligo is a very different place, and we debated that one for days before settling on an amount we felt our locals wouldn't object to. It turned out we were wrong, but I'll come to that in a moment.

Opening hours were another hot topic. Kilkenny opened its doors at 7 a.m., as many people came in to swim or use the gym before going to work, but I wasn't convinced our clientele would do that, and I didn't want to be paying staff to come in and have nothing to do. Better to open a bit later and have them busy.

And who should our staff be? What kinds of qualifications and experience should we be looking for, considering the fact that there was no real history of leisure centres for them to have worked in before? We eventually employed a manager who had run a swimming pool and took on some younger but experienced people who could learn more on the job. In that way, we could build a confident and tightly knit team, I was sure.

What classes should we provide? Which packages should we promote, and what kind of deals should we offer to the employees of local businesses? I was convinced that by tempting in a cohort from some well-known local firms, the word of mouth would get us plenty more interested parties.

I worked 18-hour days for weeks on the project, and I loved every moment of it. I was convinced the leisure centre was going to be a huge success, and prepared myself to reap the rewards of my efforts. I arrived on the day of the official opening to find a small but very vocal group of protestors at the gate. For a moment, I thought they must have come to the wrong place – this was the day we were opening our shiny new leisure centre; the hotel wasn't hosting anything else, so what could they be protesting about?

Then I got out of my car and saw their placards, and understood it was the leisure centre that was the object of their ire. And that *really* confused me. I invited the protestors inside and tried to work out what exactly the problem was. I had photographers, journalists and a guy from the local radio station coming to the opening later, and I didn't want the story to be about my group of political activists.

Well, I sat and listened to 20 minutes of a diatribe in which I was informed how we were 'changing the face of their town', courting the 'corporate collective' who were trying to 'monetise our health and wellbeing' and how the hotel should be 'a resource for everyone, regardless of the type of car they drive or whether or not they wear a tie to work.'

I let them talk, before finally getting down to brass tacks.

'You're upset about the membership fee then?' I asked.

There was a lot of humming and hawing, but what it all boiled down to was that they didn't feel they should have to pay to use the swimming pool. I had to fight hard not to laugh in their faces.

'There isn't a swimming pool in the country with a roof over it you don't have to pay to use,' I retorted, and showed them the door.

That same group protested every single new development in the town of Sligo for the next few years before falling out over something and going their separate ways. And as it happens, their leader later joined the leisure centre. I personally took his membership fee from him, and he handed it over without batting an eyelid, and without any apparent awareness of the irony of the situation.

The centre opened despite the expressions of unhappiness from that local anarchist collective and membership was fully sold out within the week. One person later laughingly told me that joining would save him a fortune, as he would not need to shower at home for the rest of the year. I considered putting savings on hot water into our future promotional materials, but in the end decided against it. That could be a hidden benefit our members could discover for themselves.

PART FOUR

Selling Ireland to the Americans

I Stop Making Sense

While working at the Sligo Park I took six weeks off in January and February to work with Fáilte Ireland, the Irish Tourist Board, as part of a sales team based in New York. Every year they organise a major promotional blitz encompassing 14 cities right across the United States. My job was a decidedly menial one: I got to organise all the brochures and marketing material in their New York office, box them up and then mail the pallets to various locations around the States. There were 80 Irish businesses taking part, which meant boxes and boxes of material needed to be sorted. This was not exactly the most exciting job in the world, but its importance was not lost on me. The cost of participating in the promotion was considerable. Each business involved had to stump up travel costs and insurance, not to mention the price of printing up all the pamphlets and flyers. If that business then arrived in Cincinnati and there were no brochures there to distribute it would be a total disaster. It was my job to make sure that didn't happen.

Once all the boxes were dispatched, I had a few days to myself to walk the iconic streets of New York. Despite having lived the first half of my life in Dublin, nothing I had seen up to this point prepared me for the sheer scale of The Big Apple. The crowds, the frenetic pace, the mind-boggling height of so many of the buildings, the roar and boom of traffic and trains. Everywhere I looked there was something I'd seen in a movie or on a TV show. It was as if I'd stepped out of reality and into a fantastic dream.

And then, of course, there was the music. During one trip I took the opportunity to visit The Power Station, the most renowned recording studio in the world in the early 1980s. All the big bands recorded there, including my beloved Roxy Music, so I was determined to see it. With a neck of brass and a determination to mine every last drop of my native Irish charm, I knocked on the studio's front door. A long-haired, bespectacled young man answered, and I informed him I was a music fan who had travelled all the way from Ireland on a kind of pilgrimage, and that he would be making all my dreams come true if he would just permit me to have a quick look around.

To my surprise and delight he grinned, and warmly invited me in to have a tour of the three studios. There was a band finishing off an album in one, and the guitarist and singer, who was a very tall and lanky guy with dark hair and the most intense eyes I'd ever seen, seemed to take a shine to me.

'Come in and see what we're doing,' he said.

I followed him into the studio and sat in the corner with my mouth tightly shut. I was expecting to hear a song, or even a guitar solo, but instead I was treated (and I use the term loosely) to clanging guitar chords, wailing notes, plectrums being drawn up and down the strings. To my mind it wasn't music, and it had neither rhythm nor structure.

I put up with it for about half an hour before deciding enough was enough and excusing myself to walk the streets some more. Only later did I realise that the band had been

Talking Heads, and the album they were mixing was *Stop Making Sense*. The tall guy who so kindly invited me in to watch him do his thing was David Byrne. I have to live in the knowledge that I was present at the birth of one of the greatest rock albums of the 1980s, and I thought it was drivel. That, dear reader, is why I'm a hotelier, not an A & R man.

A Lesson in Geography

As the weekend of the sales blitz dawned, the Fáilte Ireland team descended on the first city of the week: Chicago. My first job was to make my way down to the cage in the basement and locate the pallet of brochures, transport them to the ballroom and then distribute all the boxes to their corresponding tables.

The conference rooms of each hotel in every city were set up identically: 90 evenly spaced tables, all of which had four chairs on one side and one on the other. The representative of whichever hotel or holiday complex or leisure property would sit on one side of the table and four specially invited travel agents would sit on the other while they received a ten-minute presentation on the property or resort that table was there to promote.

The night before the first day of sales everyone attended a pre-conference party as a kind of ice breaker. I was never sure if this helped to quell the nerves of those presenting on the day or made them worse, but I loved attending. All the big names in Irish tourism were in attendance, from the Minister for Tourism to the Head of Bord Fáilte, as well as the general managers and CEOs of all the big hotel chains in the country.

My brother Francis, who had just bought The Park Hotel Kenmare, in Kerry, was also in attendance. He had got me the job as he knew everyone in Bord Fáilte and heard the position was available. He was joining the tour to promote his newly acquired hotel, and he and I always had a marvellous time together.

Everyone thinks they know Francis from the television, and the persona he presents on *At Your Service* and his other shows is, indeed, one aspect of who he is. He's a much more layered and complex person than most people realise, though, and at times can actually be extremely introspective.

However, at these dinners the other guests got Francis dialled up to maximum, and he was the life and soul of the party, telling stories from his life in the industry that had people rolling in the aisles and hooting with laughter. When dinner was finished, Francis would be the first person on the dance floor, and the last one off it.

I always loved being in his company on nights like this. He is much older than me and I didn't really know him growing up, so it was great for me to build a relationship with him as an adult, and to know him not just as a brother, but as a colleague and a friend.

Those dinners set the tone for the weeks that followed. At 8 a.m. the following morning hangovers had to be set aside as 800 travel agents bustled in for a light complimentary breakfast before receiving a presentation on Ireland from Bord Fáilte's communications officer. I remember sitting among the crowd as Enya and U2 blasted from massive speakers while images of the Cliffs of Moher and Skellig Michael played on a huge screen. It was electrifying, and really drove home to me what an amazing resource Ireland as a country is. In many ways, it sells itself.

At 9 a.m. sharp, the first of the 10-minute presentations commenced and Francis, together with all the others, sold their businesses for all they were worth. Making an impression in such an intense and pressurised environment is incredibly hard to do. Those agents saw 50 or more properties at each event, so it was essential to make it easy for them to remember you from all the others. I remember some of the sales representatives dressed in green suits; others wore red wigs and false beards. Some presented the agents with albums of slick photos in A3 folders, and still more presented them with gift hampers or bottles of 18-year-old Irish whiskey. Anything to be different.

Francis, of course, had his own ideas on how to make an impression. He arrived perfectly groomed in his trademark business suit with a few artfully taken A4 photographs of the Kerry countryside, but most importantly he brought a map of Ireland. Francis's logic was that Irish geography is not a topic Americans are hugely knowledgeable about – one of the most commonly asked questions at the sales shows was how long would it take to drive from London to Dublin: the answer being a very long time, and you would be likely to get very wet indeed.

With this in mind, Francis's presentation started with a 'where exactly we are in the world' lesson, and he kept the information on the hotel to a minimum. I soon realised he was absolutely correct. Those travel agents had already seen 100 photos of hotel bedrooms, most of which looked exactly the same. But none of the others had taken the time to show them where exactly in Ireland their hotel was situated in relation to landmarks like Cork's Blarney Stone and the English Market or Dublin Zoo.

After lunch there was another two hours of sales before we packed everything up and rushed to the airport before doing it all again the next day in another city hundreds of miles away. And that was the routine for two weeks. It was absolutely exhausting, but it was also some of the best fun I've ever had.

Quarantine Tales

Seattle followed Chicago, then San Francisco, Los Angeles, San Diego, a weekend in Orlando, then off to Miami, Dallas, Atlanta and Washington before flying back to New York.

Over the five years I was part of the Bord Fáilte team, the only part of the United States I did not get to visit was the Gulf Coast of Florida. We were scheduled to arrive in Tampa one year, and the night before the team had gone to Tony Roma's Rib Restaurant at Universal City in Los Angeles, but I had to leave because I was feeling unwell. I left before dinner was served, but woke up the following morning feeling great, and reckoned it must have just been a travel-related dicky stomach.

I got out of the bed and looked into the mirror, and to my horror discovered I was covered from head to toe in red spots. The hotel called a doctor who diagnosed 'classic chickenpox'. As this was considered a contagious disease, a serious discussion regarding the travel plans of the group had to occur with the California Department of Health Care Services.

They proposed quarantining the entire group, as our itinerary was far too extensive to be allowed to continue, given the nature of what we might be passing on to the many hundreds of people we would encounter.

I should point out that this unfortunate turn of events happened in 1991, the year America went to war with Iraq.

There was a large groundswell of opinion in Ireland that the sales trip should not happen that year, as due to the war most US citizens would probably holiday at home that summer. Many believed the trip too costly to justify under those conditions, and it was touch and go as to whether it would happen at all.

And now here I was about to bring the show to a stop and place the entire complement of travelling hoteliers and tourism gurus under 'house arrest' in LA. All the workshops, the formally invited travel agents, the multiple hotel bookings and the carefully planned air travel would have to be cancelled. Millions of pounds would be lost.

I was absolutely bereft. I felt as if my career was coming to an end before it had even gotten started. I would forever be remembered as the eejit who had sabotaged the Bord Fáilte Sales Blitz of '91 and bankrupted the Irish tourism industry. I would never live it down. Thankfully, I was saved from such an ignominious end. At the 11th hour the group was allowed to leave, though I remained locked in my bedroom at the Sheridan Universal for a week. This meant I missed the west coast of Florida, but did have the dubious pleasure of watching *Kojak*, *CHiPs*, *The Waltons* and a host of other American daytime TV on a continuous loop for seven days.

Each morning the doctor would call to make sure I was recovering, but more importantly to ensure I hadn't run wild-eyed from the hotel to infect the good people of the Golden State with my infectious pox. And they surely took the infectious nature of my complaint seriously. The housekeepers used garden rakes to remove sheets from the bed, and I was forced to hide in the bathroom while they worked on the room. Back then, it seemed a bit mad. Working on this book as I am during the third in a series of nationwide lockdowns due to the COVID-19 pandemic, it seems a little less extreme. Isn't it funny how history can teach us perspective?

A Case of Mistaken Identity

After my 'release' I caught a plane to join the group in Boston. I must have looked a sight, sporting a ten-day-old beard and covered in red craters, many of them still caked with white calamine lotion. We were staying in the Boston Park Plaza as it had an Irish connection. I arrived early, as the rest of the team was taking a long-haul flight from St Louis and weren't due to get in until early evening.

To my great surprise, there was a huge fuss made of me on arrival, the staff of the hotel falling over themselves to make sure my luggage (meagre though it was) was transported immediately to my room, and so much fawning that I didn't quite know how to react. A busboy very excitedly showed me to what I had been told was the 'Garden Suite'. After all the fanfare at reception, the room was actually a bit of a let-down: a standard room with a window overlooking a garden, but nothing out of the ordinary and certainly not a suite by any definition. It suited my needs perfectly, however, and once I'd had a quick spruce-up I took the lift down to the ballroom to get ahead of the game and set up before everyone arrived in an hour or so.

With the pamphlets and papers all delivered to their correct tables, I hurried to meet my long-lost travelling companions in the lobby, where Francis, slapping me on the back, informed me a dinner had been arranged to celebrate my newfound freedom. I was thrilled and not a little emotional about such a kind gesture, and we had a wonderful meal, during which we shared the tales of our adventures since we'd last seen each other a week ago.

Returning to my room at 11 p.m. that night, I was befuddled to see the lady who checked me in sitting on a chair at the door, clearly waiting for me with some trepidation.

'Please accept my apologies, Mr Brennan,' she said, apparently really upset, 'but I sent you to the wrong room.' I assured her this one was absolutely fine, and that no harm had been done, but she was not to be assuaged.

'I am off duty since nine, but I wanted to personally escort you to the correct room and express my regret over the mix-up.'

We walked to the end of the corridor, where there was a large set of double doors which opened onto a suite comprising three sumptuous bedrooms, a beautifully appointed sitting room, a dining room that would comfortably cater to 14 people, and outside a sliding glass panel, a garden complete with a fountain and swimming pool. It was stunning but I was now deeply confused. I was the guy who put the flyers and brochures on the tables. What was this all about? I finally decided I didn't care and ran downstairs to bring the group up for a party.

I woke up the next morning feeling a bit foggy-headed, and found a note had been pushed under my door. It was an invitation for me to meet the CEO of the hotel for breakfast. This was beginning to get decidedly strange, but I hauled myself from bed, showered, and tried to shave around the by now crusty and scabbed remnants of my chickenpox. Somewhat presentable in the best suit I had brought with me, I made my way down to the restaurant to meet the CEO, who looked decidedly surprised when I turned up.

It transpires my breakfast companion was Irish and a huge supporter of Fianna Fáil, the political party who were in government in Ireland in 1991. As I only worked for Fáilte Ireland for four to five weeks a year, I did not have a company credit card, so all my expenses were put on the main bill. When the rooming list arrived at the hotel, the CEO concluded John was a typing error, and the guest in question must be *Séamus* Brennan – who just happened to be the Minister for Tourism.

His face dropped when I arrived at the breakfast table, but to his credit he recovered quickly, we enjoyed a hearty breakfast and had a fascinating discussion about tourism. When the Fáilte Ireland highfliers arrived to the breakfast room they couldn't figure out how I – the lowest-ranking member of the team – was having breakfast with the CEO. And I never told them.

PART FIVE

Gwen

Unfinished Projects

My brain never stops working, and I'm constantly developing ideas and projects, even though many of them never happen. Gwen, my wife, comments regularly that if we achieved even 10 per cent of all the ideas I talk about pursuing we would be absurdly wealthy by now. And she's absolutely right.

For the eagle-eyed among you, yes, it's that Gwen, the girl I brought to Donegal to sell glow sticks with me. She was good enough to marry me – it's a good story, and I'll tell you it very soon. But for the moment, let's get back to those unfinished projects.

Our attic is full of plans for leisure complexes at Dublin Airport, West Coast cruises and hotel developments in Mayo, Monaghan, Cornwall and Scotland. And those are just a few, off the top of my head.

To put it in perspective for you, these are not just idle, passing thoughts or doodles on the back of beer mats. I'm talking about detailed business plans, projects I really put thought, time and energy into. I will have researched them thoroughly, spoken to people in the area to get their input and opinion, and done full costings and feasibility studies.

There could be myriad reasons why they never happened. I promise you, not on one single occasion did I just get bored and give up on them. If they did not get off the ground, there was a good reason for it, because the toil and effort put into each is considerable.

Gwen and I often debate whether we think these lost projects are a waste of time, or an experience that will stand to us. We can never decide. But it is all part of a life well lived. As I said to that woodwork teacher: better to have tried and failed than not to have tried at all. And luckily Gwen agrees with me.

Rising Tides and Red Lancias

G wen and I met in the Sligo Park Hotel. I'd love to be able to tell you a cute story about how we met, one that will make you smile and think that destiny stepped in and brought us together, but the truth just isn't like that.

Don't get me wrong – I liked her and had noticed this pretty girl coming in and out, but as I was working in the bar at the time, I felt I needed to keep a professional sheen on things, and I just treated her with the same courtesy I did all the other customers. Which was completely daft, but there you have it.

Gwen was a regular in the Sligo Park, as a gang of them socialised in the bar at the weekends. There was a particular occasion when one of her pals was throwing a party, and everyone was going. Everyone except me, because I usually worked that night, but as luck would have it the roster had changed and no one had thought to give me an invite, and I was too shy to raise the point.

Gwen seemed to grasp that I was feeling a bit left out, and feeling sorry for me, asked if I would be so good as to take her, as she didn't drive and the party was in Strandhill, a few miles outside town. I'm sure she already had a lift, but she was kind enough to pretend she didn't so I could feel like I wasn't being a sad sack.

I already knew I liked this girl, and I decided to pull out all the stops. I picked her up in a brand-spanking-new blood-red Lancia Delta, with cream leather seats. It was a stunning car, one I had spent months saving for. We went to the party and even though we both had loads of friends there, we talked all night, and when I was dropping her home, I knew I wanted to see her again.

I was extremely nervous, but as she was getting out I plucked up the courage.

'Can I take you out again?'

She paused, half-in and half-out of the car.

'When are you free next?' she asked. 'You barmen work funny hours.'

'I'm off next Sunday.'

She smiled.

'You can take me out then, if you like.'

'I would,' I said, and I think the words came out in a rush, even though I was trying to sound cool.

For our second date I drove to a beach just outside Grange in Sligo so we could go for a walk. We strolled along the sandy shore, the taste of salt on our tongues and the sand crunching underfoot, and in her company I forgot all about the time and the fact I had parked my precious car below the waterline.

As we strolled back to where I had left the Lancia several hours earlier, I spied a large crowd gathered around something, and I realised that something was my car. It was a spring tide and my beautiful vehicle was now sitting in a foot of water. Shouting an apology to Gwen, I ran at a full sprint to my waterlogged car and, climbing in, reversed it slowly out of the brine. It started without complaint. And it moved, which was good. But I knew enough about mechanics to be sure untold damage had been done. Salt water is the death knell for any internal combustion engine and the Lancia was not exactly a Sherman Tank.

On Monday, with a heavy heart, I drove to Dublin and sold the month-old car, buying a Volkswagen Golf from Ballsbridge Motors as a replacement. To say I was gutted would be an understatement.

The Lancia was gorgeous in every way: it reeked of Italian style and elegance. It was a rare model, slightly exotic, and the cream leather with the red finish was eye catching and classy. I now had a boringly reliable navy-blue Golf with a bog standard 1.4 engine. You knew what to expect, and you could be sure it wasn't going to be anything exciting. I hate being mainstream.

A Plastic Engagement Ring

We'd been dating for about a year when Gwen and I went to the Park Hotel Kenmare for a Murder Mystery weekend. It was fantastic fun, with remarkable attention to detail of a level I had not encountered before. The theme of the night was Egypt – we were brought into a story where we were a group of archaeologists excavating a cursed pyramid. During the weekend a murder takes place, and the participants have to solve the mystery. Actors dressed as normal guests infiltrated the crowd and made the whole thing come alive.

There were clues left all around the dining room and hotel, and we were also warned that different code words might be used to signify that someone knew something about the death. The actors were all amazing, and we had a wonderful experience. Neither Gwen nor I solved the mystery, but we had such an enjoyable time, we didn't mind one way or the other.

At some stage during the event Gwen came across a plastic diamond ring and, always full of devilment, she decided to wear it home as a joke. Everyone thought it was real when we arrived back to Sligo, and it took us ages to persuade them it was just a joke, and we really weren't engaged. Gwen still thought it was hilarious, though I'm not certain her parents were overly pleased at being made fools of.

The other downside was that no one knew how to react when we arrived back from Kenmare the following New Year's Day with a real diamond on Gwen's finger. This time we had to persuade everyone we actually *were* engaged. I never seem to do anything the easy way.

DREAM HOMES AND DREAM WEDDINGS

I saw the house of my dreams in the property section of the *Sunday Independent* in 1992. It was in Rathnew, Co. Wicklow, and it was gorgeous.

I had an American Express credit card, which offered a rewards system where you could get weekends away in B & Bs and guest houses, so Gwen and I went to stay in Tinakilly House for a few days, which just happened to be half a mile away from our dream home.

Now I know what you're wondering: is John thinking of leaving his beloved West of Ireland to move to Wicklow? The answer is a resounding 'No'. I loved the *design* of the house. That is what I was after. Once you have the dimensions, you can build the house of your dreams anywhere. I just needed a closer look.

In the month or so since featuring in the *Independent*, the house had been sold, and as Gwen and I pulled up outside, the new owners were actually moving in. Unperturbed, we introduced ourselves and explained the purpose of our visit. Happily, the new owners were fine about me measuring the external aspects of the property, which was what I needed to do.

The house was a Georgian hunting lodge with a bow-shaped gable, a centrally positioned front door and twin Georgian-style windows on each side. The proportions were perfect, and this might sound strange, but I thought it a very happy-looking house. The owners invited us in but I declined, as I had already designed the interior of *my* version of the house – I just needed the dimensions of the exterior: I needed the specifics of the windows, the brick detailing on the gables, the ridge height and the size of the fan light over the front door and window recesses. These may seem like small things, but together they resulted in the look I was after. I wanted to get it exactly right.

For Gwen and my first home I had designed a large open-plan hall, with a stairs leading to a majestic balcony which opened into the roof space, so the entrance was dramatic. Double doors on parliament hinges brought you into a sitting room which featured another set of smaller double doors leading to an open-plan dining room and kitchen. There would be one bedroom downstairs, while upstairs would contain a bathroom and two double bedrooms, both en suite.

I was extremely proud of the plan, which maximised every bit of space inside those four walls. It was a beautiful first home.

We commenced building and the house was finished just in time for our wedding on 26 October 1992 in the Sligo Park Hotel. We were stone broke but we both had jobs, and we now had a house and a car. Interest rates were at 16 per cent and the country was in a mess, but we were okay.

Our wedding was a great party – a celebration of friendship and togetherness. In total we had seven bands. I firmly believe that if you have great entertainment you can serve mashed banana sandwiches and still have a great party. If you have bad entertainment and great food, you will still have a disaster. We had great food *and* fantastic entertainment and, I can truthfully say, it was the best night of my life.

Foraging for Carpet

I t is hard to believe in today's world, a world where most newlyweds move into fully furnished houses, that Gwen and I moved into our artfully designed home without a single square of carpet.

As our first Christmas as husband and wife approached, Gwen became extremely irritated with having a concrete floor in our sitting room. I knew Francis was refurbishing bedrooms in his hotel in Kenmare and when I enquired, he told me I could have the off cuts if I thought I could give them a good home.

Telling my stressed wife I may have the problem sorted, I rented a van and set out to collect the best of what was not used in the hotel so it could grace our new home. I sorted through the cast-offs and found that some of the stuff that had come from the rooms was still in good condition. Soon I had more than enough to cater for all the rooms in our house and, feeling content that we would be celebrating Christmas on deep-pile floor coverings, I turned the van for home.

On leaving Kenmare I needed diesel but only had £10 to my name. Randall's Garage was right across the road from the Park and had a red diesel pump, meaning it contained fuel only to be used for agricultural machinery, as it was significantly cheaper. Selling this diesel to any other vehicle than a tractor or harvester is considered a crime. Randall's is situated directly opposite the Garda station in Kenmare, and the pump attendant insisted he could not help me out, as he would be seen and would be then liable for prosecution.

I ran back to the hotel, got the hotel van and parked it outside the Garda station, blocking their view and, feeling a bit more protected, the pump attendant happily gave me my diesel. And I commenced the long drive home to my bride with my newish carpet.

PART SIX

The Delights and Dangers of Ambition

A Boutique Hotel Almost Comes to Sligo

hile I was moving into my new home and foraging for carpeting, a friend of mine who happened to be a solicitor called and asked me to pop into his office for a chat. This was unusual – he and I usually met for a drink or a cup of coffee – so I assumed this had be something of a professional nature and was understandably intrigued.

In the early 1990s decentralisation was the buzz word in rural Ireland; many government departments that would previously have been based in Dublin were being moved to small towns all over the country, in a bid to inject employment opportunities and a much-needed economic boost.

Adding to this, Ray MacSharry was Ireland's Minister for Finance and happened to hail from Sligo. Local developers had constructed an office block in the centre of Sligo, which was intended to be used by some state agency or other, but just as whichever department it was were about to take up residence, MacSharry was promoted to Europe and local developers were left with an empty building with 32,000 square feet and no tenants.

My friend, who represented these developers, wondered if I might be able to turn this white elephant into a hotel. I jumped at the challenge.

I took up residence in the dining room at home with pens of various colours and reams of paper. I had an early model

Casio word processor complete with a state-of-the-art floppy disk drive, and I started to plan. On the positive side the building was in a great location. It was central to the town and served by roads to the front and rear. It also had lots of parking space available just down the street. A negative point that could not be ignored though was that the structure was designed to be used as office space – a hotel was the furthest thing from the architect's mind when he drew up the plans. This presented me with significant structural issues and forced me to consider a very particular style of hotel, one that had not yet made an appearance in the Ireland of the time.

What I was now looking at was a 'boutique' hotel: a small hotel typically with between 10 and 30 rooms, generally tailored to have unique selling points (USPs) focused around the specific needs of a location or demographic. Given the size of the building and its internal layout, I knew my prospective boutique needed to be bedroom based, and would offer very few meeting rooms or dining options. With this in mind I devised a 45-bedroom hotel. I factored in a breakfast room, a good-sized bar and two meeting rooms that could cater for up to 12 people.

It offered commercial and business customers a very attractive option in our region. I was delighted with my final plan. Negotiating the lease took a bit longer, but finally I was able to draw up an acceptable arrangement with a purchase option if things went as well as I hoped they would.

It is always vital to agree a purchase price at the start of a lease, as if not you will only be making the business more expensive for yourself should you end up buying it. This is a mistake I have since seen many times with businesses on *At Your Service*. I would have been ecstatically happy had storm clouds not been gathering on the horizon. News of the deal had started to leak, and I was beginning to be asked some difficult questions by my superiors in the Sligo Park. As far as I was concerned, I had nothing to report until I had signed on the dotted line, and until then I was still an employee of the Sligo Park simply working on a side project, which I had done many times before without upsetting the apple cart. There was no conflict in my mind as there was nothing signed – we were still very much at the negotiating stage.

As it happened the owners of the Sligo Park were oddly mirroring my own activities by renovating a new hotel in Dublin, which also happened to be in a superbly located building that had originally been meant for offices. The paterfamilias of the family that owned the Sligo Park was a Non-Executive Director of Jurys, a hotel less than a mile from where the new property was being developed, and, sensing a conflict of interest, he resigned from the Jurys board – but only once he had *signed the deal* to buy the new hotel. And that is a small but very important detail. He did not step away until he was sure there was a reason to do so. My insistence that I was not going to resign until I had another job to go to prompted a series of increasingly fraught confrontations in Sligo. According to the Sligo Park I was betraying an organisation that had nurtured and fostered my talents.

None of this was true, and I knew it was simply a ploy to emotionally manipulate me into either going or staying. Finally, in an offer I thought was extremely generous, I offered to vacate my position of Sales Manager for a month, during which time I would either progress with my plans for the new hotel or fail in my negotiations, and therefore return to my position, having withdrawn from the deal. I saw this proposal as a win-win for all parties. My bosses, however, did not agree, despite my pointing out the situation with the other Dublin hotel, which they informed me was completely different. Things reached an impasse, and my employment at the Sligo Park was terminated.

It was a tense stand-off in the end, during which I insisted I be escorted from the premises so no one could accuse me of taking so much as a paper clip that belonged to the hotel. I walked out carrying a stapler, which I had the receipt for in case anyone asked. It was an unfortunate way to end what had been more than a decade of happy, productive work. What this meant, of course, was that I *had* to make my new hotel happen. Because if I didn't, I was unemployed.

AMBITION

People with ambition are 10 times more valuable than people just going through the motions and doing their job. Ambition will drive you and push the business you work for forward.

I understand in hindsight that leaving the Sligo Park was one of the best things that could have happened to me, but looking back with a manager's eye, it was remarkably short-sighted of my superiors. Business is business and competition is competition, but being so desperately afraid of a talented young person striving to open a small business near you is a trait I hate to see in any employer.

I have always supported my staff when it came time for them to move on, often encouraging them to do so if I felt they might thrive and gain valuable experience elsewhere. Opening a business is not an easy task, and it requires much soul searching and contemplation. I have been in that position many times, and if I can offer someone a kind word, some hard-earned wisdom, or some encouragement then I am more than happy to do so. I genuinely love it when an employee asks my opinion on a project they are planning. It never causes me a moment of concern; in fact I see it as an expression of respect and fellowship. I also try to keep in mind that whatever business they are considering is probably going to be opened by someone sooner or later, so it's better to know the proprietors so you can work with them in an atmosphere of mutual understanding and support.

My bosses at the Sligo Park need not have worried, anyway. Despite a trojan effort on my part, the deal on the new hotel fell through and I was left unemployed, newly married and with a mortgage that needed paying. To say I was in a panic over this turn of events would be a mild understatement. I remember sitting in my dining room at home, gazing at the business plan that had just come to nought, a million thoughts whirling around in my head. That I might go and work in the Park Hotel Kenmare with my brother was not among the throng of ideas, but that didn't stop Francis from ringing and offering me a job. Nor did it stop me from accepting.

An Example for Us All

Speaking of ambition, one afternoon in 1995 I was at reception in the Park Hotel working on an idea to improve the service system in the restaurant when I got the feeling I was being watched. Looking up, I was surprised to see, not one of our guests, but instead a red-headed youngster dressed in a tee-shirt and jeans, his red hair freshly brushed and gelled in place. He obviously wanted to put his best side forward.

'Can I have a job?' he asked, before I even had a chance to utter a greeting. Which made me smile.

I probably would have put the youngster at 11, maybe 12 years of age, but he could have easily passed for younger. Nature had not seen fit to add height to his list of blessings, and the top of his head was barely visible over the counter top.

'I'm afraid I don't have anything going at the moment,' I said gently. 'Maybe come back to me in a year or so and we can talk again.'

The redhead gave me a polite bow, thanked me for my time, and left me to my work. Just as he disappeared out the front door, Francis emerged from reception.

'What did he want?' he enquired.

'He was looking for a job.'

'Did you give him one?'

Francis and I have worked together for so long, sometimes no words are required, and I gave him a look that left him in no doubt as to our young visitor's employment status.

'Go after him and give him something to do!' my older brother said urgently.

'Why?' I wanted to know. 'He's only a kid – he's not old enough to have on the staff yet! You'll have us done for child labour!'

'He's an altar boy,' Francis explained. 'I see him at Mass every single Sunday, and he's up and running to do what needs to be done before the priest even has to look at him. I'm telling you, this is a young fella we want to have working for us. Let him sweep up now, he might be running the bar in ten years' time.'

Heaving a sigh, I set aside my work and followed the redhead out onto the driveway. Luckily, he hadn't gone far. In fact, he was gazing with wide eyes at a BMW coupe belonging to one of our guests. Which gave me an idea.

'There *is* something you can do for me,' I said as I approached him.

'What's that?'

'Will you wash a car for me?'

His entire face lit up.

'I will!'

I pulled my car up to the back door of the hotel, and 10 minutes later my young charge was equipped with a bucket of warm soapy water and a sponge.

'I want to be able to see my face in it,' I said, and left him to it.

Twenty minutes later I was back in the office when I got that sense I was being watched again. Looking up, I saw my car washer standing on tiptoe before me.

'Do you have another bucket?' he wanted to know.

'I gave you one already,' I said. 'It's a saloon car, one bucket of water should do it. It's not that big!'

'No, I need it to stand on. I can't reach the roof.'

I brought him into the kitchen and found a second bucket, and before long he was back at his station, splashing away to his heart's content.

An hour later, I went to have a look at my new recruit's handiwork. Despite the added reach he managed to achieve with his bucket, there was still a streak right down the middle of the car he simply couldn't get to, but if you ignored that, he'd done a good job.

'What do I owe you?' I asked.

'Five pounds,' he informed me without hesitation.

I didn't even try not to stifle a laugh. Five pounds in 1997 would be the equivalent of about €30 in today's money, and there was no way I was giving this kid that amount of money for (more or less) washing my car.

'You must be joking!' I said. 'You're not getting a fiver for washing one car.'

'I'm sorry,' he shot back. 'I need £5.'

That gave me pause for a moment, because I could see there was something he badly wanted, and he was prepared to work for. I recognised the impulse, and I admired his determination, but that didn't change the economic reality of the situation.

'I'll give you €2,' I told him. 'And that is as high as I'm going, so don't even try to negotiate.'

Knowing he'd reached the end of the road, the tiny entrepreneur nodded, and I handed him his wages.

'What do you need the money for?' I asked him as we stood at the front door.

'Me and my little brother want to go to the County Finals,' he told me. 'A fiver will pay for both tickets and the bus.'

'Well, you're almost halfway there,' I said. 'Good luck with it.'

We were discussing the upcoming match when one of the guests, an American gentleman, came out of the hotel carrying his golf clubs, headed for the course virtually next door. He nodded and smiled at us as he passed.

'Mr Brennan,' my new friend suddenly said, 'I need to go.'

As he tore off after the American golfer, I heard him calling:

'Hey, mister, do you need a caddy?'

I knew at that moment that I hadn't needed to wish this young man luck at all. Like so many of the Kerry people, he made his own luck. When the guest walked past us on his way to his game, my young friend didn't see golf clubs, he saw the three more pounds he needed. I aspire to be like that red-haired young man in everything I do. You cannot grasp an opportunity you don't see.

Moving On

Gwen had a good job in an insurance and estate agency in Sligo. She loved her work and was excellent at it. Her employer at that time, Mr Daly, was very good to her, and I was aware I was asking a lot suggesting she leave such a good job, one she enjoyed so much. All her family lived in Sligo, too, making this an even bigger upheaval. Getting to Kenmare from Sligo required a 10-hour drive in those days, down some highly treacherous roads, so it wasn't somewhere you visited for the night.

My wife, however, did not hesitate, nor did she question the move for so much as a second. We put the house on the market, and it sold quickly. To my delight we also sold the plans to two other families, as they wanted to replicate the house in different parts of the country. I was very proud of those plans, so this was extremely gratifying.

So, our belongings packed and our hearts full of positivity, we began the drive to Kenmare. We were quartered in a townhouse that Francis owned in the centre of Kenmare, which couldn't have been more convenient. I started my time in the Park as an Assistant Manager to Tony Daly, the General Manager.

It was very different from what I was used to. To put it bluntly, the Park seemed dull and boring compared to the Sligo Park. The Park did not cater for weddings, funerals, baptisms, bar mitzvahs or any other type of get-together. Instead, it prided itself in looking after happy couples, something it did exceptionally well, but under no circumstances was it prepared to cope with a conference or double wedding, all the things that had kept me so happily busy in Sligo. It just wasn't what they did in Kenmare. This meant my role of Assistant Manager was very different from everything I was used to. In Sligo on any given day I dealt with numerous meetings, conferences, weddings and covered a daily management shift. I'm not going to pretend it wasn't manic, but I loved the challenge and the variety.

Kenmare was the direct opposite. The hotel did one thing, and it did it in painstaking detail. For the first couple of weeks, I didn't know if I could cope with the change of pace, and the days were *very* long, often commencing at eight in the morning. It was unusual for me to be home before 10 p.m. but it was the lack of excitement and activity that was getting me down, not the hours. I soon realised, though, that Kenmare is all about the guest. I may have been used to 150 guests departing every morning, guests who probably wouldn't remember much about their stay and the majority of whom I wouldn't recall either; I was now dealing with only 50, but of those it was my job to know all about them – where they came from and what they liked to do. I also had to be able to advise them on every detail of the day ahead.

That intensely focused service was totally new to me but I came to love it. Suggesting a guest might have a better experience driving the Ring of Beara, which they may never have heard of, as opposed to the Ring of Kerry, which was the very reason they came to Ireland, was a daily privilege.

The reward for this standard of care came at 5 p.m. when that guest returned, a big smile on their face, and told me in delighted tones how much they had enjoyed their day. Those 10 minutes I had given them made their day and enriched their holiday. That type of interaction is what service is all about. It is the backbone of what Francis instilled in the Park and in each person who works there. And my brother's vision has changed the way I think about this work I have dedicated my life to.

Serving a course from the left or right at dinner is a textbook standard and not a single guest will remember their waiter even did it. The conversations, the laughs and the quality of the attention you pay your guests are the things that make memories. Francis is one of the least technologically minded people I know (he still keeps folders full of menus and writes phone numbers down in notebooks) but without realising it, he foresaw the impact of social media and sites like TripAdvisor.

While many operators hate the ability of customers to express their views on public forums, I think it is far better than a star-grading system devoid of passion and feeling. Of course, you get some trolls who take pleasure in posting unreasonable reviews, but if you read through the catalogue of reviews a property has, you will usually get a fair indication of the quality of service it provides. And those reviews will also give you a flavour of the *personality* of the hotel.

I would much prefer a three-star hotel with personality than a coldly efficient five-star hotel. And it is forums, blogs and review sites that can tell you what to gravitate towards and what to avoid. Without even knowing he was doing it,

Francis future proofed us in a very clever way. He gave us a USP. And that is essential if you want to succeed.

Velux Windows and Doing Something Simple Well

Think for a moment about the Velux type of window. It's an incredibly simple concept – a way of fitting a window into the roof that is efficient, cost effective and immediately recognisable. It does exactly what the customer wants it to do, and the name of the business has become synonymous with the product – most people think Velux is a type of physical window rather than a brand name. And that is a sure-fire sign of the impact the company has had on the market.

What is really significant about them and their product though is that it has never been improved upon. I'm sure plenty have tried, but whoever designed that window got it right first time, and in so doing created something that no one has been able to better. And that level of quality is what every single person who starts a business should be setting out to achieve.

Obviously, I'm not here to present you with an advertisement for Velux windows, and rest assured they're not paying me to do so. What I do want to talk about, however, is the need to carve out your own path in business and create something no one else can copy. As I said in an earlier chapter, Master's, PhDs and 23 years of education may help but are not a guarantee of success – *you* are.

When I give talks at schools or when I'm interviewed

about my business philosophy, that is the message I try to push at every opportunity. If you're taking your first steps in business, no matter what area of industry you're attempting to enter, I encourage you, before you do anything else, to sit down and consider what it is you bring to the table that no one else has got. What is it about your personality, your skillset, your location, or even your concept, that sets it apart from everything else? It doesn't have to be a big thing, or a complicated thing – the best ideas are most often the simplest – but it needs to be something you can market as an experience or service only you can provide.

You have to remember how busy people are these days. They rush from one thing to the next, and while your business means everything to you and absorbs most of your waking moments, for your clients you are just one of 100 things they have to deal with on any given day. That is why making the few moments they spend thinking about you memorable is so important. For the hospitality industry, this becomes even more important, as long-lasting and successful businesses are those that generate return trade. If you want your hotel, your B & B or your restaurant to still be operating this time next year, you're going to need to establish good word of mouth, and a core group of clients who would like to patronise your establishment again.

When I arrived to work at the Park Hotel I found myself on a steep learning curve, because Francis had a very clear vision about what the USP of the Park was, and everyone who worked there had to be on point and absolutely clear on what was expected of them. For Francis, it was – and still is – all about establishing relationships. When you are a guest at the Park, you're not coming to stay at a standard hotel, however plush and comfortable that might be. You're visiting friends – friends who just happen to run the best hotel in the South West of Ireland.

Checking in to the Park is not like checking in anywhere else. The entire process can take up to 20 minutes, because we want to chat to each and every guest, find out about them if this is their first visit, and catch up with what has been going on in their lives if they're returning. Now, it goes without saying that if we sense someone is exhausted after travelling for hours and doesn't want to chat, we'll make sure they get settled as quickly as possible, but it is very important to us to get a sense of what they're hoping to experience during their time at the Park. So if, for example, we hear during that check-in conversation that Dad is dying for a pint of Guinness, we will make sure one is sent to his room five minutes after he goes up. These small things make a huge difference. Every member of our staff is taught to be attentive to such cues, and we expect them to be autonomous in responding to them.

I remember learning that the General Managers of one of the most iconic hotel chains in the world have a discretionary fund of $200 per guest per day. What this means is that, if a guest makes a complaint, or is unhappy, or needs a little something extra to put a bit of a shine on their stay, the manager can extend them credit of up to $200. I was asked once if we operated a similar policy, and I responded with a rapid 'No'. If one of our staff feels they need something to make a guest's stay better, they go and get it, and I trust them to make the right decision. I expect my staff to know that

Mr Murphy, who comes to stay every year in May, enjoys a particular type of whiskey, and to ensure we have it in stock for his stay. They should know that the Quigleys, a couple with seven children who choose to spend the one holiday they take every year with us, treat themselves to a romantic dinner and a special bottle of wine on the final night of their stay. I want to know every effort was made to make that last night as special and memorable for them as possible, with details like a beautiful flower arrangement, or a dessert they particularly like made to order.

There are other little things we do too that make the Park unique. For example, Francis introduced something many years ago that people comment on all the time. It's such a small consideration, but it's a great example of how a simple and virtually cost-free idea can yield dividends. You'll be amazed when you hear what it is. Kerry is all about the landscape. We are blessed with countryside that changes with the seasons in profoundly beautiful ways, and though I've lived and worked there now for many years, I still see new things every time I go for a drive. A field you've looked at a thousand times can seem fresh when you view it through the prism of a sun shower. Francis, astute as ever, understood this, and decided to make it a feature of our unique brand of hospitality.

During the night the windscreens of all the guests' cars are washed, and a note placed on their driver's door window so they'll see it as they're getting in (you should note we don't put it under the windscreen wiper, which would mean our guest would have to get back out again to retrieve it): *We took the opportunity to wash your windscreen so you can enjoy the views of the Ring of Kerry to their fullest.*

Such a simple thing, but it has received so much comment it has become something we're known for, a part of the overall experience that draws people back to us time and again. That personal touch, rooted in relationships we take time to build and sustain, is what makes us unique. And I can say with confidence that no other hotel has replicated it. In this, we have never been bettered.

Another important part of this period of my life was the arrival of my two children. Adam was born on 15 December 1997, and in true form he made a dramatic entrance, coming into the world only fifteen minutes after Gwen got to the hospital. Ruth joined our family two years later, on 20 August 1999.

It was a joyful and exciting time for Gwen and me, but I was going to work at eight o'clock in the morning (sometimes earlier if there was a delivery that needed checking) and it was a rare night indeed I was home before 10 p.m. – so I have to admit I missed a lot of my children's early milestones. But that is the life of a hotelier, and we made memories in different ways. I'll tell you about those later.

You Just Have to Be There

The problem with having a USP so rooted in an immersive experience is that you really do need to stay at the Park to fully understand it. I can try and describe what it feels like to be one of our guests all day, but you just won't get it until you've seen it for yourself.

Our word of mouth is exceptional – remember what I said about word of mouth? – and I am constantly told by new guests that they heard about us from friends who stayed and loved what we do, but they also comment on how much better the overall experience is than they expected, even after having received such glowing reviews from family or friends. That always makes me smile. We are in the business of giving people a truly memorable time.

This was brought home to me a few years back when we had an American man staying with us who had just such high expectations. I was at reception one morning when I got a call from one of our porters, asking me to go up to this gentleman's room. The moment I arrived I could tell he was unhappy. He was one of those individuals whose personality comes out to meet you, and this day it was peering out the door at me as I walked up the corridor.

I should explain that the Park Hotel Kenmare is a historic building. It is an Irish country hotel – a large one, but still an old-style country hotel for all that. Over the years we have adapted and adjusted it to meet the expectations of modern guests – Francis doubled the sizes of all the rooms, for example, in 1989 – but we believe the personality and quirks of the building all add to its charm. There are elements of the design we don't want to change – some rooms are unusual shapes, for example. We don't hide that fact: you can go on our website and see exactly what you are booking, and that is exactly as it should be. The guest I was about to meet seemed to have other ideas, however.

'Brennan, this isn't the room I booked,' he growled at me. 'I want the room I asked for – this is completely unacceptable!'

'I'm very sorry to hear that,' I said. 'Let me check with our receptionist, and I'm sure we can clear it up.'

I made a quick phone call and was able to establish within moments that this was indeed the exact room my irate guest should be in. It was also brought to my attention that we were full so had nothing else to offer. I reported this to him, as always, keeping my tones conversational and pleasant.

'This isn't the room on your website,' he insisted. 'The photographs are of somewhere completely different!'

'I can assure you that is not the case,' I said, still very friendly. 'Why don't we have a look and I can show you?'

I pulled out my phone and showed him the photos on our website of this exact room, and I walked him to the various locations where the shots had been taken, showing him that there was no trickery involved. This was the room he had seen on the website, liked, and booked.

'Alright Brennan,' he rumbled at me. 'But I want it on the record, I'm not happy.'

I once again expressed my regret, but there wasn't anything I could do about it, so I wished him a pleasant stay and went about my business. You might think I was a bit blasé about such a negative encounter, but I was conscious of the fact my grumpy guest had just arrived. I trusted the Park would work its magic in time. I saw him around the hotel for the next day or so, and I could tell the ice at the centre of him was melting. Where I had gotten glowers during that first meeting, at each subsequent encounter his demeanour towards me became more and more pleasant. On the evening of his second day with us, I was passing through the bar when I felt someone grab me. Turning, I saw it was my American friend.

'Brennan, I owe you an apology,' he said, pumping my hand. 'I get it now. I get what this place is all about. And I love it.'

He's been back five times since then. Sometimes, you just have to be there.

Losing Focus

The Park was and always will be focused on the guest – that is a given. But by the time I'd been there for a year, I knew we needed something to distinguish us from all the other similarly priced hotels on the market. I just had to work out what that was going to be.

Given the nature of the building (its size, location and history) I knew right off that adding multi-use facilities such as conference rooms and technology centres would not make sense. Much more importantly, doing so would just put the Park in the same market position as so many other hotels and we would instantly lose our market edge, which would be business suicide.

When you enter that particular space, you end up competing on price, and that is somewhere I never like to be, because price is not the same as *value*. And that is a critical distinction. An experience that is deeply rewarding can be worth any amount economically, as a pleasurable experience has no associated price. Therefore you can charge a premium because you are offering something personally rewarding. It is the difference between being guided to explore the Ring of Beara as opposed to the Ring of Kerry. And I think that says it all.

We looked at lots of different options before deciding we should develop a spa at the Park. This was a gargantuan task, and after much toing and froing, we came to the conclusion we would have to add bedrooms to justify the overall expenditure. This was a fear response. If we were going to splash out all this money on a venture we were uncertain would even work, then we had better make sure that, as part of it, we created something that would definitely net the Park more revenue. Our business heads took over from our natural instincts, and in this instance, they steered us in a direction that was completely wrong.

We were left with a plan that gave us four new north-facing bedrooms, which would be a hard sell as everyone wants their room to face south. The spa we designed was *okay*, but if I'm honest it was nothing special; it was, in fact, decidedly mediocre. In a fit of frustration, I scrapped the entire plan and wrote off the €30,000 we spent on architects. It was a comparatively cheap lesson in terms of value, in that it taught me a lesson I have never forgotten.

We lost focus. We wanted to build a spa, but instead of putting our energy and vision into building the best one our imaginations could conjure, we got distracted and decided to throw in bedrooms no one had asked for. We diluted our vision and ended up with a plan that added no value whatsoever to the hotel. It was a valuable insight to have, but it was crushing in terms of price.

There was, however, no point in crying over milk that had been spilt and was already starting to spoil. And to his eternal credit, Francis never chastised me for spending money badly. I closed the file on it and moved on, but I still had a spa to build.

PART SEVEN

Going Holistic

A Three-Letter Word

S pa is a three-letter word. Those among you with dyslexia may thank me for pointing that out, but the rest of you are probably wondering why I feel the need to state something so obvious. Well, here's why: car is a three-letter word, too.

I drive a car and telling you that simple fact tells you nothing whatsoever about the vehicle I own. It could be a Rolls Royce or a Mini (or a Lancia Delta or a Volkswagon Golf). And the word *spa* is the exact same. I could be talking about the beachfront Chiva-Som in Thailand or a leisure centre and a couple of treatment rooms in the grounds of the three-star hotel on the roundabout. As with cars, there is a universe of difference.

I knew a well-conceived, thoughtfully designed spa would suit the Park perfectly. The problem was we were a million miles from knowing what a good spa could or even should be in Ireland. Spas that featured on the 'world's best' lists were all in the Far East, in dreamy locations like Thailand and Singapore. I had no intention of trying to replicate what they offered.

I already understood I would have to create something new, and the ambience of the hotel, its location and the surrounding countryside would tell me what that something would be.

Gwen and I researched and researched but neither of us could decide what we wanted. Francis had met a lady, Susan Harmsworth, a few years earlier in Chewton Glen, in the UK, who had made a career in the spa business. I looked her up, and Gwen and I arranged to meet her during The Spa Show in London, which we hoped would give us loads of ideas for our own project. How wrong we were. The show turned out to be aimed at a target audience of hairdressers and beauty therapists and was a world removed from the kind of spa we had in mind. I was very downhearted, thinking the whole idea was turning out to be a dead loss. Nevertheless we met Susan as arranged in the Mandarin Oriental Hotel, and within the space of 10 minutes the clouds parted and the sun shone through.

Susan spoke a language that completely encapsulated what we envisaged. It was as if she could reach into our minds and pluck out the ideas. But not only that, she could expand on them and make them better. She suggested we go downstairs to visit the new spa she had just designed. It was like entering another world. The texture of light changed as you walked down a long, high-ceilinged passageway, water cascading down walls of blue granite creating a sound that was crystalline and melodic. The air smelt of jasmine and citrus, and the colours of every surface were muted yet defined. Assuring.

The staff who greeted us were relaxed but knew their craft inside out, and you sensed you were in completely safe hands. They walked us through the packages on offer and showed us to the most beautiful pool area I had ever seen to relax on recliners while we waited to be called for our treatments.

Without exaggerating, it was a transformative experience. It felt that just by being there we were becoming more relaxed. Healthier. Happier.

Gwen and I did not talk all the way back on the plane because our brains were in overdrive. We now knew exactly what we wanted. All we had to do was build it.

The House of Healing

The *Independent* newspaper printing plant had just been built on the Naas Road outside Dublin. It was a stunning example of architecture as art, a glass-walled building holding up a substantial roof and all the mechanical production equipment on view for all to see. It was fresh, modern and boasted superbly clean lines. I contacted a good friend of mine in the trade to see who had designed the building. Without pausing for breath, he was able to tell me it was Oppermann Associates, a firm of architects based in Dublin.

The second I finished the call to my friend, I rang Oppermann's offices on Foley Street and left a message. They didn't call back that day, so the following morning I rang again, once again spoke to a receptionist who informed me she would ask one of the partners to call me. I thanked her and returned to waiting.

After the fifth such call I was getting frustrated and I told the same receptionist that if the company didn't want the business I was bringing their way, that was fine. I would give them until the close of the business day to return my call, after which time I would go elsewhere. As she had done every other time, the young woman informed me she would relay my message and I hung up with little hope I would be doing business with this company after all.

So it was with some surprise that I took a call from an architect called Michele Sweeney later that day. She apologised sincerely, informing me they were 'up the walls', as it was the height of the Celtic Tiger and construction was booming so loudly it was a wonder we could hear ourselves think. I told her my vision for the building and right away she agreed to come down to Kerry with the owner, Stephen, on the first flight the following day. It had taken a week, but things were finally moving.

You may be wondering what role Francis had to play in this entire process, and the answer is very simply: he gave his consent for me to move ahead with it. Francis, as I've already mentioned, has huge talents in a vast number of areas within hospitality and business in general, but architecture, design, co-ordinating builds, choosing the types of treatments a spa might have – all these things leave him completely cold. He was very happy to allow me to take the reins, and he continues to do so on similar projects to this day. It's how our partnership works.

I picked Michele and Stephen up in Farranfore Airport, and on arriving at the hotel we walked the whole grounds and discussed various areas for the spa to be located. Stephen was anxious it be placed beside the golf course, where he felt it would balance the building and create symmetry of space, while Michele proposed it go underground in front of the restaurant, with a rear window overlooking the water.

I didn't like either option. I preferred a wooded knoll to the west beside the bedrooms. It would require excavating a considerable chunk of rock but you only have to move that once, after which you have something special for life. We agreed this was the place, though they warned me the cost of removing the stone would be expensive. The big positive for me was the build would not interfere with hotel operations. We would create a separate entrance for the builders, and all vehicles, equipment and materials could be brought in without guests seeing a scrap of it.

Another thing that attracted me to this location was that we could easily construct a tunnel entrance that would link the spa to the bedrooms as opposed to the lobby, thus eliminating the presence of dripping people in bathrobes from the main hotel. It is a pet peeve of mine to be sitting in a hotel lobby, enjoying a drink or reading a paper and suddenly someone clad in nothing but a bathrobe plonks down beside you. It's something I always feel my guests can do without. And now, it wasn't even an issue.

After a rocky start, we were up and running with a beautiful design and a perfect location. What could go wrong? Quite a lot as it happened. I was about to encounter protest again.

Differing Opinions

Building a facility like this on the grounds of such an historic building was frowned upon by some. I was told by hotel management and some of the braver members of the staff, as well as by a few guests, that I was changing the fabric of the Park forever; that I was ruining the hotel; that I was breaking with tradition; that a change so extreme was not good for such a well-established hotel. And on and on it went.

I fought my corner, but the reality was many of the dissenting voices were simply not for turning. Remembering that the ethos of the Park is wholly client-centred, I decided to go to New Jersey to meet with our most regular guest, Mr Knipper, a fine gentleman who typified our core client group. I thought he would make a good sounding board to present the project to and I wanted to see how he felt it would alter the atmosphere of his beloved home from home. I drove from New York to his home in Morristown where he sat me down in his den and listened while I outlined my plans for the spa, explaining the location, the benefits I hoped it would bring and the reasoning behind its creation in the first place – the concept that the Park needed to move with the times and carve out a niche for itself in the rapidly evolving world of hospitality.

To my horror I got the same reaction: change is not always good; the Park has a certain ambience the guests treasure;

what about the fine tradition Francis had established over many years? I was gutted. Why was I doing this when the world was against me and no one seemed to want a spa in the Park? I was ready to write the whole thing off for a second time and just sit back and let the hotel sink or swim based on its existing merits. I don't get downhearted often, but this was beginning to feel like a fight I couldn't win.

On the flight home I met a very well-connected Dublin business person. They were familiar with spas around the world, and I was pleased to hear they knew of the Park, though they had never been to it.

'Do you mind my asking why not?' I enquired.

'You're just not on my radar,' was the response.

'Can you tell me why, though?' I pressed.

My travelling companion thought about that.

'I would say your hotel doesn't speak to me,' was the answer. 'You're old, traditional ...'

'Stale,' I finished the sentence for them. And that summed it up perfectly.

The evolving market of clients who used hotels regularly were not interested in what we offered, and we were losing business and market share as a result. At that time we were still closed five months of the year, which was an absurd reality. Francis, while wanting to encourage my creativity, was becoming very worried that my work would impact on the integrity of the hotel in a negative way.

But I was now convinced I had to act, and soon. If something didn't change, the Park did not have a long-term future. Which meant I had to force that change to happen, whether my colleagues – and my brother – wanted it or not.

MEN TO THE RIGHT, WOMEN TO THE LEFT

I got off that plane convinced the spa was the right thing to do despite all the opposition. Now we just had to decide what we wanted it to be.

The Sheraton Hotel in Edinburgh probably still has the greatest offering of thermal rooms in any hotel. I went to have a look, and found they offered 15 in all: laconium, rock sauna, crystal steam, ice fountain, experience showers, Turkish bath, floatation bath, and on and on. I thought I had best try them all out to see what I was dealing with and, resplendent in my Speedos, I began my circuit.

The laconium suite (a dry heat room, invented by the Romans) was the first on my list, and when I went in I discovered two ladies seated inside having a chat. I thought this was fortuitous, and thought I'd join them and ask what aspects of the spa they enjoyed the most, which ones they didn't like and if they had any suggestions for my project.

I needn't have bothered. They left within 30 seconds of my arrival.

It made me think about something Mr Knipper had said to me in New Jersey during my disappointing visit:

'John, I will never go into a room full of strangers wearing nothing but my togs, especially if those strangers are women.'

Those fleeing ladies had just proven his point. They had been having their weekly get together and I had inadvertently invaded their space. There and then I decided we needed two thermal areas, one male and one female. This would, of course, double the costs, but would make for a vastly better experience. It is a feature many have commented on as being unique and extremely welcome. And I have Mr Knipper and those two ladies to thank for it.

We applied for planning permission and I was certain it would be approved but at the last minute an objection was logged on the basis of the Park being a protected structure. The spa, according to the objector, was an inappropriate development. I was beginning to think protestors would plague me for the rest of my life, and I was furious as we had spoken to all our neighbours and no one had raised an eyebrow, never mind an objection. It turned out the unhappy individual was not even from Kenmare and had nothing to do with the area. As far as I was concerned this was a nuisance objection, and I relished the process of having it thrown out.

SÁMAS

With such an investment we needed to get our marketing right. Francis traditionally looked after all the marketing at the Park, but we needed new eyes for this as we were hoping to break into new markets. From our days in America with Bord Fáilte we had come to admire a lady named Margaret Ryan, who had been Director of Marketing for Ryan Hotels at the time. She was now freelancing, and came to visit and see what we were doing. We clicked instantly – she just understood what we were trying to achieve. It was the beginning of a long relationship. Rarely a day passes where I don't exchange at least 15 phone calls and as many emails with Margaret, including Sundays. I don't know what I'd do without her.

The next job was to find a suitable name for our new spa. I felt it needed to belong to the place; that the name should reflect the very fabric of the earth it was hewn into. Because we were taking 15,000 cubic meters of rock from the ground we came up with 'Strata'. I liked the idea, but the word seemed too cold and masculine. I knew we were on to something though.

Twenty million years ago Kenmare was the location of a massive earthquake. As the limestone bedrock was pushed to the surface, a sea of lava washed it into the sea, where it formed an underwater shelf called Mellon House Coral. To this day Kenmare town sits on a layer of limestone while the surrounding area is all sandstone.

I thought 'The Mellon House Spa' was a perfect name: exotic and a bit tropical, it also presented us with a great marketing story which spoke of the very foundations of Kenmare Town. I was sure we had it, but a voice in my head told me to road test the name before printing up any business cards. It was a good thing I did. The first English guests I spoke to burst out laughing the moment I told them the name.

'It's like you're calling it "The Boob Spa"!' one woman told me between shrieks of laughter. So that name had to be abandoned too.

There was nothing left for me to do but go to the library, a place I was never in before or since, where I researched Irish names. Close to the back of the Irish/English dictionary I came across the word *samhas* which translates as 'indulgence of the senses'. It was perfect except for the challenge of pronunciation for anyone unused to the vagaries of the Irish language. I had visions of Americans asking me what exactly 'Sam Has' for the spa to be named after him. And it would invite word play, particularly with the male and female thermal suites: 'Sam Has' and 'Sam Has Not'. That would drive me mad.

We were close, but still no cigar. It annoyed me for days and over the following weekend Gwen and I joined our friends Michael and Maureen Hayes for dinner. As I was telling them the story Maureen, a schoolteacher, solved the problem in one fell swoop.

'Drop the *h* and add a *buailte* (a dot) over the *m* and you have the traditional Irish spelling before the letter *h* was even added to the language,' she said. 'It's much more authentic and will be easy to spell and remember.'

To celebrate we ordered another bottle of wine. As I sipped a glass of Tokaji, I realised something else: in its new form the word was now a palindrome, perfect for a reflective spa. SÁMAS was born.

A Second Case of Mistaken Identity

Coordinating the building of the spa was an absurdly complex task in itself, involving a series of almost daily site meetings. Architects, engineers, quantity surveyors, builders and subbies all needed to be consulted and directed. The team was enormous as the complexities of thermal rooms, water treatment plants, air handling, light management, wall coverings, fittings and 101 other things only intensified as the job progressed.

At one meeting the question was raised regarding the process of joining the glass panels to the roof. Much discussion took place around the dangers of weathering before I asked Michele from Opperman's how it was done on the *Independent* newspaper building that had been the inspiration for the whole build. Michele went quiet for a moment before admitting her company had not a single thing to do with the *Independent* building.

My friend had got his information wrong all those months ago, and either Michele and her associates didn't realise I was labouring under the impression their artistic vision was behind the *Independent* building, or they just decided it would be better not to tell me otherwise. I was floored. We were in the middle of a multi-million-euro build and I had never seen a single building my architect had designed. But it was too late to do anything about it, so I chose to see it as a lesson rather than a problem. Always check your facts!

After a 13-month build SÁMAS opened to much fanfare in May 2003, gracing the covers of *Condé Nast Traveller* and *The World's Top 25 Spas*, a success in itself. The Park Hotel Kenmare had just entered a new world.

If Susan Harmsworth, founder of the iconic ESPA brand, was considered the mother of spas, Bernard Burt would be considered their grandfather. He owned a very small travel agency in New York called Spa Finder, which has now become an online portal for finding spas the world over, and he was coming to Ireland on holiday. I needed to get him to Kenmare. After much wooing and the promise to arrange his transport and look after him completely during his stay, I succeeded, and his first comment on seeing SÁMAS was:

'I don't understand why you've got no swimming pool.'

I tried to explain that, in Ireland, if we built a swimming pool we would end up with what we call a leisure centre, which is a very different thing.

'Bernard,' I said, 'in the United States you have good weather, country clubs and your kids are used to swimming. In Ireland we don't, and if I built a swimming pool the place would end up looking like Butlin's. Kids would be tossing beach balls at one another and teenagers would be doing cannonballs into the water and it would be the furthest thing from relaxing you could imagine.'

I don't think he understood. But he did say that, apart from the absence of a pool it was one of the best-planned and most fulfilling spas he had ever visited. And that was high praise indeed.

—

PART EIGHT

Retreating to Move Forward

Rooftop Gardens

SÁMAS brought the Park into a new market, which is just as I had hoped. Ireland was booming and we boomed with it. These were exhilarating times, and it felt as if there was nothing we couldn't achieve if we put our minds to it.

Shortly after opening the spa a couple came to stay with us. I had never heard of them, but they arrived by helicopter, so I assumed they were movers and shakers in whatever spheres they travelled in. That said, they were no fuss, so I got on about my day and forgot they were there. The following morning the gentleman asked to see me. Such requests usually mean complaints: low water pressure in the room; didn't like his dinner; found the bed uncomfortable; or any of a thousand similar gripes. We are, however, in the business of creating comfort, so it is my duty to listen to any and all criticisms, and try to improve on them, so I went along prepared to do just that. The man introduced himself as Sean Mulryan, and informed me with a beaming smile that he loved our spa.

'I'd like to ask you a few questions,' he said.

I said I'd be happy to chat to him, so we went to the lounge and he explained he was planning a development in the UK and wanted to incorporate a spa into it. I walked him through the ups and downs of our journey when creating SÁMAS, and he seemed very interested and attentive. We spoke for an hour or so, shook hands and I did not think of him again until I was in Dublin a week later, and received a call from reception informing me that a Mr Mulryan had booked four twin rooms and a double for the night.

I immediately flew into a rage, convinced this guy was bringing his team over to examine the spa and steal all my ideas. I informed my team that no tours of the spa were allowed and absolutely no photos were permitted to be taken in there: this is a policy we have always had, and still do – it's hardly relaxing and healing to have crowds of hoteliers or spa developers wandering about snapping photos and discussing thermal options while you have your treatment.

I got a speeding ticket on the drive home and arrived dishevelled at the hotel to be told they had all arrived and were in their rooms. And rather than being in the company of a group of designers and executives, Mr Mulryan was treating his mother and her friends to a night away to celebrate her birthday. I will never forget how I felt. I had jumped to the worst possible conclusion, and I still feel guilty about it. Sorry, Sean!

During his visit Sean asked me to join the team working on his new development. I jumped at the chance, and within the month commenced a fortnightly commute each Tuesday to Canary Wharf in London. Pan Peninsula was being developed by Sean's company, Ballymore, and a spa was a major part of the attraction. It was a wonderful experience for me, as the design team included the renowned architects Skidmore, Owings & Merrill, who were behind many buildings I greatly admired, like the Al Sharq Tower in Dubai.

The spa was situated on the fifth floor overlooking the flat roof of the entrance overhang. I wanted to open the windows of the vitality pool onto that roof and create a garden atop it that would be breathtaking on a summer's day and would offer a reason for people from further afield to visit the spa – an oasis in the centre of London's business district.

Skidmore, Owings & Merrill did not share my vision, however, stating that it would detract from the clean lines of the building. They were right from an architectural point of view, but those lines added nothing to the users of the spa, and I very much doubt they drew any customers. I still think it was an opportunity missed. I relished the project, as it was on a scale the like of which I had never had the opportunity to see before, and with professionals at a level I had never gotten close to. Secretly though, I struggled to see who their client base was going to be.

Building the Perfect Retreat

The hotel was flourishing, and I was restless for something new, for a fresh idea to inspire me. I had just taken on a serious challenge and come out on top. Getting SÁMAS off the ground had been massively difficult, but not only had I done it, I'd created something that set a world-class standard of excellence.

I didn't have to wait for long. We had a 24-bedroom apartment block that had traditionally been used as staff accommodation, but as houses to let began to appear all over Kenmare the need for accommodation for staff in the hotel became less of an issue. Rather than using the accommodation on site, our staff generally preferred to rent a house together in the town, leaving the staff block sitting idle.

I spent a few weeks tossing around ideas as to what we might do with the space, and finally decided we should build a residential development dedicated to providing a heightened living experience for the owner rather than a typical hotel holiday home development. As you are aware by now, I hate being typical.

I researched the international market and was amazed to find very few hotels with dedicated residential development. They all seemed to opt for the rental option – some did offer long-term leases, but the numbers that chose to go down the residential route were negligible. I thought about the reasons for that and continued my research. It seemed that all the hotels with resident-only apartments were city based, and the apartments in question tended to be purchased for private use as a second home. That is what I wanted but in reverse.

The trump card we held was we had the best of both worlds: our hotel was moments from Kenmare town centre, while effectively also being in the country. Would we find people looking for such a situation? I strongly believed we would. In fact, the more I thought about it, the more convinced I was this was a good bet.

After the success of the spa I had no hesitation in engaging Oppermann Associates again. The design we hit upon for the block was that all apartments should have an identical layout: two bedrooms with ensuite bathrooms, an open-plan living room/dining room/kitchen opening to a south-facing balcony, a TV room and a wine cellar and basement store. Each apartment would come with two car parking spaces.

I reasoned that two bedrooms would be perfect to suit retired owners, giving them the option to entertain another couple on occasion. Plans were agreed for a total of 18 apartments, 18 storerooms and 36 car parking spaces. The beauty of the design Oppermann drew up was that while the apartment block would look like one building, it would in fact be three identical buildings connected. This feature meant we could place two apartments on each landing, so the owners would only have one neighbour, making the whole project very private and discreet. Now we just needed to add the coup de grâce. And this was going to be a swimming pool.

During my work on the spa at the Pan Peninsula I had worked with a company based in Sweden that specialised in stainless-steel pools. While these are three times the price of a conventional pool they require much less maintenance, have a far longer life and the water quality is considerably easier to treat, using fewer chemicals and therefore avoiding that unpleasant chlorine smell so many pools have. I had found the company wonderful to work with, so we invited them to Kenmare to view what we had planned. This was by now the third swimming pool I had been involved in, and my experience taught me that pools in hotels tend not to be true swimming pools at all. They are designed by architects to look nice and have the 'wow' factor, but for swimmers the odd shapes they tend to have make doing laps impossible, so they did not fulfil their function.

SÁMAS and all its facilities was built for the guests at our hotel, but the pool was designed for owners of the apartments. This was a bold decision, but it reflects our commitment to offering unique and tailored experiences to both our residents and our guests. We planned a 25-metre even-depth swimming pool, a glass-walled sauna and an experience shower – one with water effects like tropical rain or cold waterfall – to add some thermal facilities to the space. The Park was finally going to get its swimming pool.

The Tender Art of Tendering

With the fine points decided, the tendering process began. There was a local builder who wanted to tender when I was building the spa, but I was forced to refuse as while they were local, they were far too young and inexperienced. The spa was a complex build, and although I admired their ambition, I did not feel they were ready, and I wasn't prepared to absorb the risk.

When this fledgling company heard of our plans for the pool and apartment block the owners, Brian Gallivan and Donald Lynch, approached me again to request a chance to tender. I was happier now, as they were more experienced and had completed a number of well-finished developments. Added to this, they were local, and hungry for opportunity.

When the final tenders had all been submitted KPH, the local company, had made us an offer €10,000 below the next lowest, which was from the construction giant Sisk. This put me in a quandary. John Sisk is a good friend and regular guest at the hotel. All his children got married with us, exceptions are made when they visit, and he and I share a passion for boats.

Tender tradition has it that you invite tenders from companies you are genuinely prepared to do business with, and the rules of engagement are that you must take the lowest tender. However, with only €10,000 in the difference the two lower bids were deemed equal and the design team all favoured Sisk. They had the experience, I was reminded, a highly skilled team and a head office with expert contacts all over the world should the project run into difficulties. In other words, Sisk came with the sure-fire ability to pull off what was going to be a complicated and very technical job; one that required a high-quality finish.

On the other hand, we had KPH, who I knew had the passion and commitment but not the history or experience. It was a Catch-22 situation. The design team was nervous, because they sensed I was leaning towards employing the local crew. And in the end, in spite of vocal opposition, I appointed KPH and work commenced in September 2006.

The first job those local lads had to tackle was to remove 30,000 cubic metres of rock, which took months. The land in the Park Hotel Kenmare seemed determined to never yield easily to development. But we persevered, nonetheless.

For the apartments to meet the increasingly high standards of the market, they needed to be really special. I commissioned David Linley from London to design a show apartment. His classic lines, meticulous attention to detail, and colour palette finish was perfect, and he really set the look for what we decided to call The Retreats at the Park Hotel Kenmare. Bringing him on board was a decision I have never regretted, and his work continues to inspire me.

KPH pushed forward with the ground works and The Retreats began to elicit enquiries from prospective buyers just off the plans. I was tempted, but I resisted making any sales until the show apartment was finished. As the building progressed, I ordered Linley furniture for the show apartment, and that sense of luxury and opulence really began to take shape. The finished living space had nine-foot-high doors, shadow-line skirting, floor-to-ceiling windows and no corridors – I hate corridors, as they are a pure waste of space. Every bedroom had recessed lighting, sliding pocket doors and beautiful bathrooms. I knew we were on to a winner, as nothing like this existed anywhere else. Yet again, we had created something unique, a living experience that could not be bettered.

Know Your Audience

Some of the first people I showed the show apartment to were Leslie and Carmel Buckley. They had been good friends for many years and were regulars at the hotel. They, in my mind, typified the profile of potential buyers. When the viewing was complete I asked them the burning question:

'Would you be interested?'

Leslie's response knocked me for six.

'If I was 30 years younger I'd take it in a flash. But John, we already have our second home.'

I realised there and then that I had misjudged who our potential residents were, and lo and behold the first people to buy an apartment in The Retreats were a couple in their forties with two young children and a dog to follow. They were not at all who I had envisaged when I conceived of the project, but I couldn't have been happier to sell them the most gorgeous apartment in the development right off the plans, as the building was nearing completion.

I was elated that we had made our first sale and felt that new and interesting things were just around the corner. In 2007, Ireland was the fastest-growing economy in Europe. Companies were shipping staff in from overseas because there were so many jobs to fill. The property market was booming and the tourism trade was growing massively year on year.

The future never looked so positive, and I was excited to see what it would bring.

Little did I know it was bringing one of the darkest periods of my career, a time when I wondered whether everything I had worked for was going to come crashing down. And it all began with a financial services firm named Lehman Brothers Holdings Inc.

PART NINE

The Dark Times

The Bubble Bursts

What always amazes me is that none of us saw it coming. We probably should have done, because all the signs were there, but I have to tell you, hand on heart, I was as blind-sided as anyone when the Irish economy imploded in 2008.

There had been rumblings, and the Irish Central Bank warned us in March of 2007 that the level of consumer borrowing was unsustainable, but this announcement was followed by the then Minister for Finance, Brian Cowen, advising us through a radio interview to continue right on as we were – there was, he claimed, nothing to be concerned about. The Irish economy, he stated, had never been healthier. And God love us, we all believed him. Me included.

But Ireland doesn't exist in a vacuum, and events taking place on the world stage were about to overwhelm us. Lehman Brothers Holdings, a massively influential global financial services firm which had exerted a major influence over the markets since its inception in 1847, had been investing heavily in sub-prime mortgages – mortgages given to people with very low credit ratings, meaning they are high risk.

Such a huge company should have known better, but the gamble did not pay off, and the United States Federal Reserve went in to try and arrange finance for the company, summoning a number of banks to provide the capital. The negotiations floundered, and on Monday 15 September 2008

Lehman Brothers filed for bankruptcy. The impact of this single action was catastrophic.

That night the Dow Jones stock market index closed with a drop of 500 points – the biggest fall in its history, exceeding even the drop following 11 September 2001. But things were to get worse, and on 29 September there was an even greater slump, driving the markets down further.

Just remember, most of the Kenmare Park's guests came to us from the United States, meaning an economic recession there was going to hit our hotel business very hard. But that was only the beginning. The problem internationally was that so many other financial institutions were exposed to Lehman. Major companies in Canada, Japan, Germany and the UK all went into freefall. The Royal Bank of Scotland alone lost $1.8 billion dollars in unsecured loans to the company, a loss that took them years to recoup.

In Ireland Anglo Irish Bank was the worst-affected bank, but there were other dangerous financial dealings going on behind closed doors no one could have foreseen. Irish banks were borrowing abroad to fund the property boom, and they were borrowing on a three-month rollover basis – effectively, this meant they had to pay back what they had borrowed at the end of a three-month period. You don't need me to tell you it takes much longer than three months to build and sell a development.

To service their loans, the banks were taking money from other funds while they waited for sales to occur, sales that often didn't materialise for several years. The entire financial system was built on aspiration – which is a tenuous kind of mortar, and not always very durable.

In 2007, the Central Bank warned that the Irish economy was becoming overheated, due to huge property developments happening all over the country – remember when the skyline of every town and city in the country offered a panoramic view of cranes and construction machinery?

Usually when a market becomes saturated with a single product (in this case property), prices go down, but that didn't happen. Instead, the price of property sky-rocketed, massaged by the developers and the media alike so that (and this is not an exaggeration) a tiny, single-roomed stone shed in a field in County Meath was advertised in the property supplement of a national newspaper at an asking price of €130,000.

It was unsustainable. The building continued, but a small population can only purchase so many properties. By the end of 2008, the Irish people had bought as much as they wanted, and the buying frenzy came to a halt, meaning the banks had nothing to pay back all those short-term loans they had taken out. And what had started out as an economic recession turned into a depression.

The banks had to be bailed out by the government, and a series of austerity budgets brought hiked taxes and increased income levies, which affected not just property but tourism, motoring and every other recreational or 'luxury' industry. Construction and property development companies all over the country went into liquidation, countless people lost their jobs and many more emigrated.

It was devastating. And this was the Ireland – and indeed the world – into which I was proposing to sell a block of luxury apartments. It's a good thing I like a challenge.

What Goes Up Must Come Down

I n the beginning, I thought we might be okay. We had plenty of viewings, multiple follow ups and no shortage of interest. But what we didn't have were any more sales. We issued contracts to five people who told us they were going to buy, but all were returned unsigned.

The property bubble had burst, the world's economy was in a nosedive and no one was buying anything. With a serious recession looming I had to admit that the timing of The Retreats could not have been worse. Before launching the project we didn't have a single bank loan. Thinking we were on to a sure thing we took a gamble, and that gamble had proven to be foolhardy.

Now our future, the fate of the hotel and all its loyal staff were hanging in the balance. The news informed anyone brave enough to listen that the banks were calling in loans left, right and centre and we must have been high on their list of potential targets. But I was not going to allow that frightening call to come.

I have a policy when it comes to dealings with banks: always keep the dialogue open. Let them know every step of the way how things are going, and whatever you do, keep making payments, even if those payments are only a drop in the ocean compared to what you owe.

To their credit, Bank of Ireland never tried to make things difficult for us. It was always me calling the meeting with them so I could outline exactly how things were progressing with us. The news, during these lean years, was usually bad, but I delivered it anyway and tried to put as positive a spin on it as I could.

A few years passed, we sold an apartment here and an apartment there and the funds the sales generated just about kept the bank off our backs. I knew by now there was no way in hell we were ever going to pay off the loan, and a haircut on a debt of this magnitude was not something Bank of Ireland would consider. I wouldn't say I was desperate, but I wasn't far off it.

By the January of 2012 I needed a sale badly. There was a couple who had looked at an apartment, showed some interest but had never followed up. Their names were Fergal and Rachael Naughton, and I had found them to be warm-hearted and honest people. I needed to pull a rabbit out of a hat fast, so I decided to be bold and give them a call. I got an overseas ringtone, but I persisted. I needed this. In fact, I needed it badly.

Finally Fergal picked up. After the usual niceties I came to the point: were they going to buy one of the apartments? I offered Fergal a very attractive price, better than what I had first quoted them, and then I held my breath.

'I'll tell you what,' he said. 'Why don't you come and see me next week when I'm home? Maybe we can come to an arrangement.' I duly went to Dublin as Fergal requested, and to my gratitude and delight we shook hands on a deal for not one but two apartments. I could feel the blood flowing again in my veins. We would live to fight another day.

Rescue Plans

The money from those sales gave us a lifeline, but the black cloud was always overhead and it wasn't getting any less ominous in colour.

The most interesting thing about the sale was the profile of resident was again not what we had envisaged – for a second time we had sold to a couple in early middle-age with children, rather than older buyers on the brink of retirement. It was another lesson: deal in what you know and bring in the experts for what you don't.

By 2012 the hotel business was slowly starting to improve. Business had dropped by more than 50 per cent during 2008 and into 2009, which was a crushing blow, but the intervening years had seen very small improvements. Yet it wasn't enough; in fact, it wasn't even close. The debts we had accrued in The Retreats were like millstones around our necks, and no matter how I turned it over in my head, there was only one way out. I was not going to sit back and allow that phone call to happen, the one where I was informed our loans were being called in.

So in 2013, with a heavy heart, I took a deep breath and followed the only course of action left open to me, and prepared to sell the Park Hotel Kenmare. Francis and I discussed the dreadful prospect, but we both knew we were staring down the barrel of a gun, and that there was no other option available to us.

I would approach the bank with a single cash settlement, in the hopes of negotiating a reduction on the figure we owed. I was confident they would go for it, as it meant they would accrue something from their investment. Letting us go under would gain them nothing.

My first port of call was a very well-known and successful Irish businessman, someone with interests across a wide range of markets. He was interested and made an offer, but the figure he presented me with was so far below the outstanding loan it left me speechless.

I had no option though but to present the offer to the bank; it was not met with enthusiasm. In fact, the bank was surprised I had decided to follow this plan of action in the first place, for a number of reasons. The hotel was again trading well, and while we weren't paying off the capital on the loans, we were covering the interest. The bank suggested we hold firm and make every effort to sell the remaining apartments, which would not even come close to paying back the debt but would put us *almost* into the black again.

Yet this plan left me with a bad taste in my mouth. We would still be in debt, and there was no certainty in the current economic climate. The hotel business was still not back to where it had been, and what guarantee did we have that things wouldn't take a downturn again? How could I, in all good conscience, sell apartments to good people with a promise of a certain quality of life, only to have to turn around in six or seven years' time and sell the hotel out from under them? I just couldn't do it.

The bank was annoyed, and I knew it, but I was not going to compromise my ideals, even in the face of financial ruin.

If you start doing things you don't fundamentally believe in, you're on a slippery slope. Francis and I have always been completely ethical in our business dealings, and I was damned if I was going to abandon my personal code now. I knew, leaving that meeting, that it was only a matter of time now. The banks were getting the really big clients off their books first, but after that their rheumy gaze would turn on businesses in our fiscal bracket. And when that happened, it would be too late to save anything.

We struggled through to September 2016. In the intervening months I purposely did not sell even one more apartment. I could not look someone in the eye and tell utter lies about the future I was supposed to be selling them. My business was spiralling towards its end, but at least I could sleep at night. Maybe not particularly restfully, but I had a clear conscience.

One Monday morning I got a call from the bank requesting that I attend a meeting in their western offices. It was the first meeting they ever called me to and I knew the time had come. Putting my best game face on, I rallied the troops. My team would be made up of Francis (who came very begrudgingly, because he hates these sort of things), our two accountants and Margaret, who was by now my administrative officer and knew the business at every level.

We arrived in Killarney and met the new area account manager – a young man from Dublin – together with our local, Limerick-based managers. I was prepared for a battle, but in the end it was more of a skirmish. I laid out the situation and our thinking on it in as plain a language as I could, after which the accountants restated it using the kind of economic jargon that makes my eyes glaze over, but seems to make bankers feel they are speaking to like-minded people.

They listened politely, but I knew they were just waiting for us to stop talking so they could deliver the ultimatum we all knew was coming. And it was quite the sledgehammer blow in the end. We were told in no uncertain terms that if we did not have the hotel sold by Christmas, the bank would take it. I could sense Francis trembling beside me, and I didn't know whether it was anger or sadness. I thought it was probably equal measures of both.

'What about our Personal Guarantees?' he asked the new official from Dublin.

Francis was referring to legal guarantees Francis and I had signed over the loans, assuring us of a certain standard of conduct from all parties involved. The new man from Dublin smiled at my brother indulgently.

'If you assist us in the sale of the hotel, we would look on such considerations favourably,' he said condescendingly.

Francis tensed visibly.

'What does "favourably" mean?' he demanded.

The bank official began to outline a litany of considerations and possible scenarios, none of which offered my brother nor I any comfort, and I could see him shrinking in upon himself as the full horror of what might be happening dawned on him.

That's when I saw red.

'Excuse me,' I interjected. 'You're new, so I'm going to give you a bit of leeway, but I think it's very important I explain one or two things to you.'

The new boy stopped in mid-sentence, his mouth still open.

'I am an *employee* of the Park Hotel,' I said, my voice betraying none of the annoyance I was feeling. 'I am not a shareholder and neither am I an investor. The Park pays me a wage, end of story.'

He started to speak but I raised a hand and ploughed on.

'My wife owns Dromquinna Manor, a property situated just three miles from the Park Hotel Kenmare. If the bank forces a sale of the Park, I will hand in my resignation immediately, as is my right, and I will reopen as the Park at Dromquinna.'

(I'll fill you in on Dromquinna later on – it's an amazing story.)

I could see the Dublin official's eyes widening. I had him on the ropes.

'And let me promise you this,' I concluded. 'There will be no goodwill for your version of the Park, and absolutely no good publicity. I'll make certain of it.'

I stood, and the others followed suit. We shook hands, but everyone in that room knew the first shots of the war had been fired, and it would not be long before the second volley sounded.

Shock Tactics

I t was a bad time, one that might have been made easier if Francis and I sat down and talked things over, but in truth, we didn't. It wasn't that there was bad feeling between us, it was just that we were too weary. I think we were both in shock. And in that shock, we froze.

Francis had spent his whole life building the hotel from nothing, and now it looked as if all that work was going to be *for* nothing. I may have taken the gamble on the apartments, but my brother was also caught up in bad investments, so he knew he bore an equal portion of responsibility for the position we were in.

I didn't ever point the finger of blame at him and he never lost his temper with me. It would have been so easy to give vent to all the anger and hurt and resentment and despair. But instead, we just didn't talk about it.

We each had houses, loans, commitments, reputations – and I had a young family, too. The future was uncertain, frightening, and I feared things might get very messy before it was all over.

With no cards left to play I phoned the man who had put an offer on the hotel some years previously to see if he was still interested. As luck would have it he was, and would be in Dublin on Saturday, so I arranged for Francis and me to call to his home for a meeting.

The meeting offered us a sliver of light in the tunnel. I spent the days before the meeting compiling figures I thought the bank would accept. If I could get this deal right, it just might work for everyone. I whispered a silent prayer and put the papers and notes that would, ultimately, facilitate the handing over of the Park Hotel Kenmare to a new owner, into a folder. Now all I could do was wait.

Two days before I was to drive to Dublin for the fateful meeting my phone rang. It was Fergal Naughton, he who had bought the two apartments in 2012. He was calling from Australia but would be home in two days and was planning on coming to Kenmare.

'Can you turn on the heat for us?'

I was in the first of his apartments doing just that when a thought struck me like a bolt from the blue. Maybe this gentleman could be an investor – meaning he would buy a share in the hotel, take a chunk of the equity, and get the bank off our backs all in one go. I phoned him back and asked if he might spare me five minutes on Friday evening. Accommodating as ever, he said he'd be happy to give me ten.

It took me a little longer than that to explain the information to Fergal and Rachael and to lay out all the figures, and when I did, he was far from certain he wanted to be involved.

'The numbers are huge,' he told me earnestly.

'Believe me, I know that,' I said ruefully.

'And you're meeting the other guy tomorrow?'

'Tomorrow morning, yes.'

He shook his head and sat back.

'I'll tell you what John,' he said. 'Do nothing until you hear from me. I need to think this over and make some calls.'

I was on the road to Dublin when Fergal phoned, and to my delight said he was in, but wanted to meet me again before making a formal agreement. Which left me with a dilemma. Here I was on my way to meet someone who wanted to buy everything, but whose offer, I was sure, would still leave a burden on our shoulders with the bank. Should I turn the car around and do a deal which I hoped would leave Francis and me some equity in the hotel, and free us of bankers for good?

After a few uncertain moments I decided to keep driving, as having two irons in the fire was always better than one. Knowing I had a backup plan, I was more confident during the Dublin meeting, putting forward figures that would leave us in a stronger position. The businessman seemed happy with my projections, and asked us to give him until Monday evening.

Francis and I thanked him and drove back to Kenmare as if the hounds of hell were chasing us. I went to Fergal and Rachael's apartment alone, as Francis had had quite enough at this stage, and said he'd trust me to make the right decision.

Rachael, who is a solicitor, opened the discussion by telling me she had two questions: Firstly, was Francis happy with the idea of going with them? This was a lovely question, as it demonstrated they knew the connection Francis had with the hotel, and I told them Francis would be more than happy so long as he kept his reputation and could continue doing the thing he loved.

The second question brought a smile to my face, because it demonstrated just how astute Rachael was. She wanted to know what condition the roof of the hotel was in. It was a brilliant question. The Park Hotel Kenmare dates from

1897. If the roof was no good, it would cost millions to replace. Luckily, I could report it was in excellent condition, as we were very conscientious in maintaining it. These two questions answered satisfactorily, the agreement was made. We shook hands there and then, and I went to tell Francis we were home and clear. It was an emotional conversation.

This meant I was able to inform the businessman that I would not be entering into a deal with him – and that I was able to make a very satisfying phone call to the bank. I phoned the Bank of Ireland offices in Limerick at 10 a.m. on Monday morning and asked, 'If I walked into the bank with a cheque for X would the bank be prepared to close the file on the Park and wipe the Personal Guarantees?'

'John, I think if you walked in with that, they might even be prepared to bring you for lunch,' was the answer. I made damn sure they did, too.

I owe Fergal and Rachael Naughton a debt of gratitude I will never be able to repay. They saved the Park Hotel Kenmare from disaster on two occasions, and have proven to be wonderful partners and great friends.

Looking back on it, I have to say I find it inspirational that, during those most dreaded of years, amid all the anguish and gloom, Francis and I managed to find hope and friendship. There are many businesses I know of that fell under the weight of that terrible recession and many people who never recovered from the pressure they experienced. And I do wonder if the stress took its toll on me; but before we get to that episode in my life, I've another story to share with you.

PART TEN

At Your Service

An Unwilling TV Star

Let's back up a bit. In fact, let's go right back to before the dark times. Let's return to 2007, when Ireland was riding high and on the crest of the economic wave. Anything seemed possible, and opportunities I would never have thought plausible five years earlier were suddenly coming out of the woodwork unexpectedly.

Francis did a one-off TV house renovation programme which had gone down well, and he was approached to consider a hospitality mentoring show for RTÉ, Ireland's national broadcaster.

Francis has a very unique style and flair, and an easy way with people. He has a great eye for design and is extremely articulate, able to communicate difficult ideas and complicated strategies in simple but effective language. He is an ideal host for a TV show, and the camera loves him. My brother loves both film and theatre and has an almost encyclopaedic knowledge of both. He brings this with him into each show he is involved with, adding his own ideas to how episodes should be structured, the tone, themes, messages and stories that can be told within whatever the genre of the show is embracing. You might think it's just a property renovation, but alongside the story of how the building is transformed, you are also watching a human journey. Francis is acutely aware of that.

I have never been able to understand why the makers felt it would be good if I was involved, but I got a call from Maggi Gibson, a producer with Waddell Media. We made an appointment to meet in Dublin for a chat.

What people often don't realise is that Dublin in those days was a seven-hour drive from Kenmare: literally a two-day excursion. You didn't just 'pop up' for a cup of coffee. If I was travelling, I always did my best to pack in a few other meetings to make the trip worthwhile. And the truth was, I had absolutely no interest in launching myself on a TV career – frankly, I needed it like a hole in the head. I had so much going on at that stage in my life, all of them projects that interested and excited me, that I just wasn't invested in a prospective TV show that might never reach the airwaves anyway. Maggi had been nice on the phone though, and a voice in my head told me that if nothing was ventured, nothing could be gained.

In 2007 the iPhone was still a thing of the future, so diaries existed only on paper. My own personal planner was always cluttered with densely written scribbles (scribbles put there by a dyslexic, to boot) and I forgot all about the meeting. In fact, I never even went to Dublin. The afternoon I had arranged to meet her I received a message in the hotel that someone called Maggi was looking for me. I felt bad but reckoned she must have at least 100 other interviews with people she might team Francis up with, so decided I wouldn't be missed. And I didn't call her back.

The following day I got another message. For someone whom I had stood up and not returned calls, Maggi was very understanding and forgiving, and we made another appointment in Dublin for the following week. Seven busy days followed, and lo and behold, I forgot all about the meeting yet again.

I know I'm coming off as very rude here, and I suppose that's fair. In my defence, though, if I'm interested in something, I will prioritise it and make it my business to make things happen. The problem here was I was very definitely *not* interested. And when Maggi called me this time to ask why I hadn't shown up for our meeting, I told her so. I had neither the interest nor the time, and she would be better placed to find someone else. Maggi tried to sell me on the idea over the phone, and I had to tell her as plainly as I could that while I was an ambitious person, none of that drive was to be on the television or to be famous. Such things didn't hold any allure for me.

Maggi was not going to be easily dissuaded though, and over the next couple of weeks more calls and letters arrived – the producers believed the dynamic between myself and Francis, two brothers who had worked closely with each other for years, would be a great selling point for the show. Could I just spare her one hour so she could pitch her idea for the show to me?

I told her about the challenges of getting to Dublin, but she had an answer for that. Waddell was based in Belfast, and at the time there was a daily flight from Belfast to Cork. Maggi suggested she could come to Cork to meet if I would agree to go that far. I had to admit it was very generous of her, and as I had been so rude, I thought I had better make amends, so we made an appointment to meet in the Old Victoria Hotel the following week. This time I wrote the date and time on Post-it notes and stuck them everywhere so I could not possibly miss *this* meeting.

Screen Testing at the Old Victoria

Cork is only a 90-minute drive from Kenmare, and on any given day I'll have countless things to do there, so even if the meeting came to nothing it wouldn't be a wasted journey. And Francis and I had some history with the Old Victoria.

The hotel in question is a city-centre-based hotel that had originally been located over a Burgerland (these were very popular fast food outlets in Cork, though they aren't around anymore). Straight after leaving college Francis worked there for a time and during his tenure I stayed quite a bit. My brother rapidly rose to the level of Assistant Manager at the Victoria, and with his help the hotel made its mark as the best in Cork.

As the place really got into its stride Francis's boss at the Old Victoria had to take sick leave for a prolonged period, which left my brother in the unofficial role of General Manager (though he was never given the title). It was an amazing experience, but he was still only getting the salary of an Assistant Manager, which his superiors were reluctant to increase because of his young age – he was only 25 at the time.

The manager did not return, and when Francis forced the issue, insisting they either promote him to acting GM or he would leave, they called his bluff. Except it wasn't a bluff, and my brother walked.

What management at the Old Victoria didn't know was that during this time Francis had been approached by Mr Weeland, who wanted him to go to the Park Hotel Kenmare, which he had just bought, to take up the position of General Manager there. Francis had refused, hoping he would resolve things in the Old Victoria, but on the day he walked out the planets must have been aligned because Mr Weeland was sitting in the lounge having coffee. Francis literally strolled from a meeting in which he had just handed in his notice right into another impromptu one in which he was given a brand-new job within the space of 60 seconds. And the rest, as they say, is history. So it felt a little bit auspicious having a meeting about a brand-new project in this hotel that had been so pivotal in my and Francis's career.

Maggi met me in the lobby and we chatted about hotels, hospitality and life in general. I had since discovered I was the only one in consideration for the position, and on the two occasions we were to meet in Dublin the producer had travelled to see me especially. It made me feel like a total prima donna – behaviour I would consider absolutely horrible in anyone else. I apologised profusely and made a silent vow to try and make it up to Maggi.

A bedroom in the hotel had been booked, as Waddell needed me to do a screen test. I didn't even know what a screen test was, but Maggi informed me that the majority of people look, feel and speak differently on screen. TV audiences watch a film or TV show and form an opinion of the person they are watching, but what they are actually seeing is a persona that is created by the producers and editors of the show and is rarely any reflection of what that person is actually like.

I know this now from personal experience, and I have to tell you, once you have worked in that world you will never view anything you see on a screen in the same way again. Working in TV ended up ruining TV for me. Which might not be a bad thing, if you really think about it.

Anyway, the plan was for me to walk into the room where there was already a cameraman in place recording everything. Without acknowledging the camera's presence, I was to point out and explain which aspects of the room were commendable, and which I saw as problematic. They would film it all in a bid to establish whether or not I *worked* on screen.

The Old Victoria was a very different hotel from when Francis worked there. In 2007 it was quite dilapidated and in need of a lot of tender loving care. It was, if you pardon the expression, one of those hotels where you would flush the toilet with your foot, a foot that was clad in sturdy boots, because no one was going to walk on any of the surfaces in their bare feet. You get the picture.

The first thing I noticed on arriving at the door to the room was that it had been fitted with a Yale lock, which is a sure sign everything had been done on the cheap. There is just something unsatisfactory about a Yale lock on a hotel bedroom door. Don't get me wrong, Yale make a fantastic lock and I have many of them in properties I own, but never on a hotel bedroom door.

You want to establish that a guest is entering somewhere special, somewhere out of the ordinary, right from the beginning. Unlocking their door using a key-card, hearing those tumblers whirring as if by magic, is an experience they won't get at home. Chances are lots of rooms in their houses, and possibly even their front door has a Yale lock. A terrible start.

The door itself was one of those white doors with four white panels and close to 100 coats of paint applied by a bad painter. It had a tarnished brass handle picked from the bargain basement of the local hardware store and the threshold was worn and scuffed. I hadn't even opened the door yet, and already I was appalled. Taking a deep breath, I pushed the door open and immediately burst into guffaws of involuntary laughter. Maggi screamed:

'Cut! Cut! Cut!'

But I couldn't stop. The reason for my mirth was that the curtains and the upholstery on the room's chair were made from a material patterned in an American-Indian ethnic style. It was a material I recognised immediately, as my parents had it in their house in Sligo.

'What's wrong?' Maggi wanted to know, but I was beyond answering at this stage. I had lost all composure.

The material was so unusual only one thing could have happened: when Francis left the Old Victoria in the late 1970s he was owed a lot of money. I had to imagine that as he was planning his exit strategy, the rooms were being renovated and he decided to take a roll of material with him in part payment – which had ended up in the curtains and furniture in my parents' house in Sligo. It was not like the Francis I knew, but I reckoned he must have been more ruthless in the heady days of his twenties. It was the only plausible conclusion.

Having composed myself (and making a mental note to give Francis an unmerciful slagging) I re-entered the room and did my screen test, making a few surreptitious comments about the soft furnishing that Francis would pick up if he saw the recording, but which no one else would see as out of the ordinary. I assumed my brother would watch, and would know I'd discovered his 'crime'.

We wrapped and, satisfied I had fulfilled my obligations to Maggi, I departed for Kenmare. I hoped that would be the end of my adventures in television.

A week later Maggi phoned to say RTÉ liked the test and would be delighted if I took part in the show. I was speechless. Well actually, one word did spring to mind, a slightly more aggressive version of the word 'feck'. You know, the one with the 'u' in the place of the 'e'.

I needed an excuse and I needed one fast. The only credible one I could think of, and in fact it really was the truth, was that I just did not have the time to spare. There was the Park, the Retreats and my consultancy practice. There just wasn't room for a TV show in among all that. I was sorry, but I was going to have to decline.

'We can make it work,' Maggi said.

This was not what I wanted to hear. I decided there and then to lay my situation out for her as starkly as I could. I could not commit to leaving Kenmare for lengthy periods of time. Francis and I had not really spoken about the project in depth, but from the brief conversation we did have, I knew the filming schedule would require my being away for several weeks if I was to fully commit. I just could not give that time investment.

Maggi, however, was not for turning. A format was created where Francis would visit a struggling hotel, B & B or guest house, assess the situation and then phone me to discuss what should be done. There would be a camera crew with me in Kenmare and one on the road with Francis to capture both sides of the conversation.

And so the first series of *At Your Service* was filmed and broadcast on 4 September 2008, just as the world collapsed. In an act of bitter irony, the recession and the lack of business it engendered meant I had much more time to devote to my burgeoning television career. While the work I loved was shrivelling on the vine, a job I had neither asked for nor wanted became the thing I am best known for. Sometimes life plays tricks on us. Not that I was laughing.

The 'Why Nots' vs the 'Why Bothers'

During Season One of *At Your Service* I managed to escape Kenmare to visit three of the eight properties featured. It was a very strange experience to walk into a business you know absolutely nothing about, hear the owners' stories, examine their work practices and running procedures and then give them advice.

In keeping with our personal ethics, I was adamant that nothing about the show was to be done just for the sake of TV audiences. We were not doing this just for the sake of making a TV show, we were doing it to help the people who appeared in the show, and also those viewing.

I always held the belief that someone with a struggling business might be watching and get some ideas that could set them on a path to turning their situation around. This is a very different approach to many reality-based TV programmes, where the host is the star and the other participants little more than props. I made it clear that I would not do anything I did not believe would work or be good for the business long term.

We were coming into a business, poking our noses into the owners' lives and we never wanted to give advice just to improve the content of the show at the cost of the business. We wanted to walk away at the end of shooting believing that, if the family we had just worked with carried out all the instructions we had given they would have a better business. If they didn't? Well, that was their problem. At least we had been honest and done our best. And that is as much as anyone can aspire towards.

Of course, I am now aware that some of the more compelling shows across the series were where our 'owners of the week' *didn't* take our advice and the viewer is sitting at home, shouting at the TV: *'What's wrong with you?'* After one such show I got a call from a friend saying she was 'breathing into a brown paper bag by the end'. But that is the nature of the medium. Conflict and tension make excellent components for an exciting story. Though they can be very frustrating when you're a part of that story.

The first season was scheduled to air on a Thursday evening at 8.30 p.m., a very desirable prime-time slot for an unknown show. Francis and I waited with bated breath. We didn't know what to expect. For the first show I hadn't been able to visit, so I was only shown speaking to Francis on the phone from Kenmare – Francis was very much the star of this one. But it was a good show – pacy, well edited and funny, and Francis's interactions with the family and their guests was charming and authentic.

The reaction from the press and the viewing public was overwhelmingly positive. People loved the format of the show. They loved Francis and his flamboyant, colourful style. They even loved me – I was seen as the 'money guy', Francis's slightly more serious and edgy younger brother whom he called to deliver the bad news or crunch the numbers. Which is not me at all, but remember what I said about TV creating a persona?

As the other seven episodes in that first season aired, two common threads began to emerge. Ninety per cent of the problems facing the owners we tried to help stemmed from two types of situations. There were the 'sunny day dreamers' – people who visit a location in the summer months when the place is swamped with tourists, think it is beautiful and buy a property, never realising how bleak it will look in the depths of November when there isn't a soul about and the rain is coming down in sheets. Then there were the inheritors – people with neither the skills nor the inclination to learn who had inherited a guest house from a relative.

The other thing that really surprised me was our audience profile: we had viewers ranging from aged six to over ninety years of age. *At Your Service* was perfect family viewing. As soon as that first show aired, we would have kids coming to the hotel asking us questions like:

'Why did they not do what you told them to?' or 'Would they not have made more money if they changed that?'

We had countless questions like that. I love that young people watched the show and hope some of them will be inspired to get involved in business. I think the kids who watched picked up on the ideas, the problem-solving and the potential of the different locations we visited. The youngsters I have spoken to all got that the show is about the capacity to change. Adults tended to view it more from a voyeuristic point of view – look at the mess this crowd are in!

It might be a generational thing. A 12-year-old looks at a challenge, comes up with a solution and asks: 'Why not?', while a 40-year-old sees the same situation and wonders: 'Why bother?' Despite my age I still respond like a youngster. Which is a much more positive, if stressful, place to be.

The Sunny Day Dreamers – So You Think You Can Run a B & B?

Have you ever heard someone (maybe you've done it yourself) criticise a café, restaurant or hotel? It doesn't matter what the cause of your complaint was – it might be anything. I want you to think about it for a moment though. Your criticism was based on your opinion.

Opinion is the easiest thing in the world to have, and your opinion on how that café is running its business is rarely tested. No one expects you to have the skills to step behind the counter and put your ideas in motion to see if they would help that establishment perform better. If everyone who complained or voiced their distaste was expected to do that, I think the vast majority of such constructive critiquing of businesses would cease immediately, which would be a shame. It's why opposition politics is a much safer and easier place to be than in government.

Many, many people we encountered on *At Your Service* were individuals who had spent years telling themselves they could run a particular style of hospitality-based business better than all the others they had encountered. Coming into some money, or perhaps using their savings, they finally bit the bullet and bought somewhere, usually in a location they'd visited, and thought was idyllic. These are the sunny day dreamers, and they had no idea what they were getting themselves into. The various seasons of *At Your Service* were riddled with them.

Let me give you an example. Take a small business, a B & B, for instance. Here is what the couple think as they buy the property: 'We have four good-sized bedrooms. The hotel down the road does a lot of weddings and the area is busy with tourists, so we should have no shortage of guests. If we were booked to capacity six months out of the year we should make €80,000 per annum.'

The couple think of this in the same way they would a regular wage. They may even see it as cash in hand, and open their B & B. The reality is very different indeed.

First off there are the logistics. One room is departing at seven in the morning for a flight and they want breakfast to go. The owner has to be up and at the cooker at six to get that ready, but the other room are on their holiday and want a full Irish breakfast at ten, as late as possible. They go out for the day and you make all the beds, wash the sheets from the room that has just departed and while you're doing all that you also have to be available to answer the door and the phone to take reservations or walk ins.

Your new guests arrive at 3 p.m. and would murder a cup of tea and slice of cake. The tourists arrive back after a great day and are full of chat and expect you to spend time hearing all about their excursions and to be interested and engaged (the fact you've been up since the crack of dawn washing, cooking and taking reservations never even enters their heads).

Another room arrives to check in and, as they are going to a wedding they drop bags and run to the celebrations. They are totally flustered because her hair appointment went all wrong and they were late departing, so they aren't in the best of moods and are curt and ill-tempered. At 11 p.m. the tourists arrive back from the pub and bang doors, talk loudly and start a singsong in the sitting room as the fire smoulders. At 4 a.m. the wedding couple return and cannot remember what room they are in. That's assuming they can find the house and you aren't woken by them ringing you to ask what the address of the place is. You have to get ready and help them, and you must do so with a smile on your face, despite the fact they are blind drunk. You finally get them to their rooms but at some stage he goes to the toilet and misses. That will be waiting for you to clean up when they leave.

Breakfast the next morning brings a whole new set of problems. The new arrivals had an awful night between the tourists banging the door and the couple returning from the wedding. They were in the next room and the walls are as thin as paper. No one caught a wink of sleep. They are silent and sullen and when the door opens to the breakfast room and a couple walk in no one makes eye contact, because everyone is annoyed at everyone else (and there is probably a degree of embarrassment at play, too).

You return with the fry and say a cheerful 'hello' but the atmosphere is tense and you realise you'd be better off not bothering. Both depart, and one leaves a comment in the Guest Book:

Nice house, great hospitality, bad mattress, cold bathroom, thin walls lots of noise!!!!!!

It is 11.30 by now, and there is no sign of the wedding couple. You knock on the door and get a grunt. At midday they arrive down with bloodshot eyes looking for coffee.

Their bags are only half-packed and one of the lads has his shirt buttoned up incorrectly as they make their way out the door. You are happy to see the back of them.

The phone rings. It is a reservation for two couples going to a wedding in November. It's a good way off, but it *is* €240, so you can't really say no. You take the booking and go upstairs to clean the recently vacated room of your wedding goers. The bed is soiled, the bathroom is an unsanitary mess and the curtain rail has been pulled from the wall.

Downstairs the post has just arrived with a collection of official-looking envelopes: bills for oil and gas, electricity, the phone, Booking.com and an invoice looking for the annual fee from Fáilte Ireland. The HSE would like to arrange an inspection, and you also have an invoice for the local cash and carry for your washing powder, breakfast cereals and bread. This collection of good news is rounded out with a letter from the Local Community Association looking for sponsorship, as you must be making a fortune.

At some stage you have time for a coffee with the other half, who has just fixed the curtain pole in the bedroom, and he tells you he can't go to town to look for new sheets as rain is coming and the grass needs cutting.

Five years pass, and the excitement of opening your dream business has worn off. The €80,000 a year you expected has turned out to be closer to €10,000 when all bills and taxes are paid. And you have no life. You are exhausted and the dream is dead.

Most of the cases we tried to help on *At Your Service* had loans they could not pay and were looking down the barrel of a gun held by the bankers. They were at the point where they couldn't see the wood for the trees and were too caught up in operations. Most had given up living and were drawn and exhausted – old before their time.

The life of a small business owner can be horrible. No one ever decided to open a bad restaurant, but we have all eaten in them. The reality is that talking about something and actually doing it are very different things. Knowing how to run a business and being able to do that well is key to success, and that is one of the main problems we encountered with *At Your Service.*

Having opinions about what a B & B *should* be like is very different from having the actual skills to put that into action. It is a great industry and I love it, but enter it young or with your eyes wide open. It is not for the fainthearted.

Inheritance – Don't Bequeath a Life Sentence

Of all the things to bequeath your children, do not give them a life sentence. If they are genuinely interested and have a good grounding in your business, then that is a great legacy to inherit. If they don't and are only involved because you built up the business and they feel indebted, then sell the thing and let them do as you did and start something *they* are passionate about.

I have seen too many owners in their sixties struggling to keep a business together because it is the family heirloom. They don't have the skills, personality, vision or drive to make it work. They are at an age when they should be enjoying retirement and have no money and their lives are filled with struggle, unhappiness and stress.

Why? Because they were given something they should never have received. In many cases, where the business struggles, it is the member of the family who is the most shy and retiring who inherited the business. Why? Because the others had followed their dreams and poor old Harry, who never pushed himself or his needs forward, got the business because he was still at home.

Some of the places we visited still stand out in my memory. Often for all the wrong reasons. I have looked places over during our initial assessment, and subsequently refused to sleep there, because the rooms were so damp and dirty I would rather sleep in the car, which I did on many occasions. I have moved dinners we were served to show us what culinary marvels the owners could produce from one side of the plate to the other because they were inedible. I have looked at owners (who had agreed for us to come to make the show) and seen total disengagement in their eyes.

On other occasions we have arrived with the team for filming to find the owners gone on holiday. I've never been able to work out if they were running away from us or just totally disinterested when that happens. And I'm not sure which is worse.

On another show, one which proved particularly popular, a young son was taking over his family's business and a lot of money had been invested. I thought he was a great young guy, full of positive energy and ambition. Left to his own devices I was sure he would be a huge success, but he was encumbered by external factors in the form of two siblings who didn't want to be on TV themselves but wanted their opinion included in just about every scene we shot, exerting their influence from behind the camera.

They would stand behind the cameraman and 'observe' everything their brother said, obviously making sure he was reflecting whichever message they wished to have conveyed. Twenty minutes after Maggi called 'cut' he would ask if the piece could be filmed again, as he wanted to change what he had said.

No decision on any aspect of the business could be made, as each time we sat down to discuss options the lad's mother, father and two siblings all began vying for dominance, yet it was clear to me from the start that the son was the only one going to make it work and, more importantly, was the only one willing to try. And he was becoming seriously stressed by the constant squabbling and backbiting. It was a state of affairs that Francis and I were unable to rectify – we were there to try and improve the business, and the course of action we proposed was sound and would certainly have yielded positive results if followed. The problem was, though, that they did not need two business advisors. They needed a therapist and a family mediator.

The business struggles today, and I genuinely fear for that wonderful young man's future. Inheritance is a cornerstone of the problems he continues to face. He inherited the family business, but along with it he inherited a family dynamic that simply did not work, and that dysfunction spilled over and infected how the business was run. I believe the best, and indeed the kindest course of action, would be for them to sell the business, divide the proceeds and allow that young man to strike out on his own, unhindered. He might open a café rather than a hotel, but he would make a success of it without being encumbered by all that family baggage.

Making Television

We normally film *At Your Service* with just one camera. The first reaction is always focused on the owners. So when we film a scene the camera will be aimed at the owner, we say what we have to say and then the camera moves to behind the owner and films us repeating the question or giving our opinion.

I have never liked this, as two cameras are far better because both moments are captured simultaneously. To me it is very obvious the interaction was cut and the pieces just don't flow as they should because, in reality we are repeating what we said or did just moments before and it is never the same delivery.

Of course, the viewer doesn't see it, but I do. Maggi always assures me it is a technique that works, and it is true that no one has ever complained, but it is just not as natural as it could be.

At one location I was delivering the crushing line:

'You have two choices: close today or go bankrupt in September.'

It was a horrible ultimatum to give. I was 40 years old at the time, and the man whose life I was devastating was 65. And I was telling him his dream was over. That the 40-year journey he had been on was wasted and everything he had laboured for had come to nought. You only get to deliver that line once, and both reactions needed to be captured in unison. I insisted we use two cameras and the entire (very moving) scene was captured to perfection.

But of course, we didn't always come to a location to rain on their parade and deliver bad news. There were many, many places I would be happy to revisit as a guest, and many owners I have kept in touch with. Francis and I were often inspired by the enthusiasm and drive we encountered, and these owners' love for what they do jumped off the screen – their businesses blossoming as a result – because the viewers liked what they saw and wanted to support them.

Success is created from the fusion of commitment, knowledge, vision and noble effort. And the beautiful truth is that success breeds success. Francis and I saw that first hand with *At Your Service*.

The show pulled us through the challenges of the recession as it attracted top ratings and, while our colleagues and competitors were forced to spend money they didn't have on advertising, we were on TV morning, noon and night through this new role neither of us ever envisaged or planned. Francis's personality was infectious, and the Park benefitted as a result.

By Season Three we had secured the coveted 8.30 p.m. slot on Sunday night, and had been feted on *Tubridy Tonight*, *The Late Late Show* and every talk radio show in the country. Francis, who discovered he had a personality for TV presenting, started doing other shows, and did a string of very popular travel shows to boot. The world, it seemed, was our oyster. And such amazing success brought wonderful blessings. But it came with some curses, too.

The Price of Having a Well-Known Face

The huge popularity of *At Your Service* allowed us to think bigger. As the seasons passed, we started to bring owners to well-established hotels and hospitality businesses to show them what best practice looked like. We did this in the hopes they would recognise things they were missing and carry these lessons back home. I am a firm believer that travel and seeing something first-hand is far more educational than any book. At least it is for my dyslexic brain.

You might think this totally self-indulgent conceit, but I justify it by reminding myself that spending a weekend in a luxury hotel that costs upwards of 30 per cent more than a place that is simply nice will probably teach me something new that I can then apply. It is also very important to see what new choices and experiences your guests could have and analyse what you are doing compared to the competition.

Getting out of your daily routine, even for a day, can be life changing. I find that small businesses get so caught up in the grind of daily operations that years can pass and a particular way of doing something can become entrenched. Before you know it, you are behind the times and out of touch with market trends. If you don't get out and experience the market, you will never know if your business is keeping pace with it.

So bringing owners away from their properties and their particular corners of Ireland proved a wonderful addition to the show. It brought the viewer on a journey too, and introduced fresh elements and new landscapes and locations. I'm also proud to say that countless new friendships were created between the owners and the people who ran the places we brought them to, the majority of which are still blossoming today.

The ability (and the money) to take our owners of the week on these excursions was a wonderful benefit of our success. But that success came at a cost, too. A personal one. And if I had known about the price, I never would have agreed to do the TV show at all. *At Your Service* is a peculiarly Irish show, and has not found an audience anywhere else. So when I say we have a successful prime-time series, I am speaking purely in Irish terrestrial viewership. But in Ireland, I am now famous, or to put it another way, everyone knows the show, and once that first show was broadcast, my life changed instantly.

Before 4 September 2008 I only knew people who knew me. These relationships occurred naturally and were developed as a result of the bonds of family, work, hobbies and shared interests. It was reciprocal – anyone I interacted with knew a little bit about me and I about them.

With TV success all that changed. Everyone suddenly thought they knew me, though I did not have a clue who they were. It is one of the weirdest feelings. I think this aspect of the show has particularly impacted on me because, unlike lots of people in the media, I never craved a public profile.

I remember going down Henry Street in Kenmare one night

with a couple who are very well known. I spotted someone in a restaurant who is a friend, and told my famous companion I was just popping in to say 'Hello'. To my amazement the celebrity I was with asked: 'Would you like me to say hello to them too?' I didn't know what to say. I thought it was such an odd suggestion to make. Why would you put yourself in a position to be mobbed – which is exactly what happened? Luckily I had a particular table booked in Packies, a restaurant in Kenmare that is now unfortunately closed, which I chose specially because it is situated in such a way that you can see the whole dining room but no one can see you. Martin, the proprietor and chef, always booked Table 1 for me and it was the best table in Kenmare – of course apart from all my tables. On this occasion it was perfect as this couple have no peace when they're out.

As a result of the show if I want to eat in McDonald's, I use the drive-thru and eat in the car, because if I sit at a table inside, within five minutes, someone will approach me asking me what I think of the food, and how many stars I'd give it (even though we don't give stars on *At Your Service*). I don't enjoy the constant intrusion, and I hate being rude to people, so I find it is easier just not to bother.

I am not saying public-profile people are divas or that they possess massive egos. What I am saying is that they have a life in the media that dictates public interaction and attention. They knew they were taking that on when they chose that career, and being a public persona is their job. It is not mine. I had a wholly separate career long before *At Your Service*, and I was very happy in that world. In truth, it was a world I had no desire to leave.

The struggle I face is how to remain in it, while also inhabiting the world of (sort of) celebrity. It is a Catch-22, as you cannot have a successful TV show without the loss of privacy.

So You Want to be a TV Star?

A good friend and regular guest of the hotel came to me once for some advice. I was somewhat taken aback to be asked, as this person is at the top of their game and internationally revered as an expert in their field. The BBC had approached him to do a TV show in the UK in the same mould as *At Your Service* but instead focusing on the retail trade.

My friend was delighted to be asked, and I thought his personality, which is down-to-earth, warm and approachable but 10,000 per cent professional would jump off the screen. The show, I had no doubt, would be a resounding success, and would bring all kinds of opportunity my friend's way, given the reach of the BBC. That said, the gentleman in question is not a public person. He likes nothing more than to sit at Table 3 in our lounge on his own and read a paper over a pot of tea. He comes to the Park to unwind, and for him that means quiet solitude.

Over the course of a lengthy conversation, I asked him why he was considering doing it. His reply resonated with me, because it reminded me of the rationale I had when I embarked upon Season One of *At Your Service*. He told me he wanted to give something back.

I responded by asking if he was happy. Did he want for anything? Did he have any unachieved goals? He immediately told me that he was extremely content, and wanted for nothing whatsoever. We had known each other for many years, and I asked why he thought I didn't spend much time in the lounge at the Park anymore. He shrugged and told me he didn't know, but I could tell he was starting to understand.

I told him Gwen had gone shopping in Cork the previous day, but hadn't wanted me to go with her because I would slow things down. Or at least, the constant interruptions from people wanting to say hello, pose with me for pictures and asking for advice on their own business dilemmas would.

My friend listened intently as I told him about how Brad Pitt, the Hollywood actor, wanted to take his kids on a train journey from London to Scotland to see their mother, who was filming there. His goal was for his kids to have the experience of seeing the landscape change as they moved out of the urban sprawl into the countryside and then again as they reached the highland in a proper locomotive, a mode of transport not availed of very much in the United States where they lived. It was a genuinely English thing to do, and Brad wanted the kids to experience it.

Unfortunately, Mr Pitt understood that they would see almost none of this on a normal passenger train, as the entire trip would be taken up by fans, onlookers and journalists looking for his and his children's attention, making it a complete waste of time and not the special experience he wanted them to have. In the end, he rented a train so they could do the trip in peace.

Back in the Park my friend nodded and, reaching over, shook my hand.

'I think I've made my decision,' he told me.

'I thought you wanted to give something back,' I reminded him.

'There are lots of ways I can do that,' he said. 'Ways that don't involve giving up life as I know it.'

There is a wonderful song by Joni Mitchell called 'Big Yellow Taxi'. In the bridge to the chorus she sings about never knowing what you have until it's gone. I had just saved my friend from that fate, and as a result he can still enjoy reading the paper over an uninterrupted coffee at Table 3.

PART ELEVEN

Bed Factories

An Offer I Can't Refuse

During this time another guest of the hotel asked to see me, offering a chance to be involved in an interesting project. Seán Dunne was a Dublin-based developer who had stayed with us a few times and had once asked us to host a party for his wife's birthday. I don't mind admitting I was watching him surreptitiously, as he was all over the news for buying Jurys, The Towers and the Berkeley Court Hotels in Dublin at a record price. I met him in Ireland's capital in early September 2007, and over lunch he set me a challenge.

'I want to redevelop those sites but it will take time,' he said. 'The team I have working on it are saying it could be a year or more before we'll be able to break ground.'

I nodded sympathetically, although I was privately thinking his team were being very optimistic in their projections.

'Here's what I'm thinking,' he said. 'Business has never been better than it is now, and I know I'm losing money having those three buildings sitting there gathering dust. I'd like to open them for a limited time period – say, a year, perhaps, maybe 18 months, to see what kind of income they can generate. And I want you to do it.'

I tried to play it cool, but inside I was jumping up and down like a child who had just been given the keys to the local toy shop. Each of the properties was in a prime location, they were all in immaculate condition, and between them had a total of more than 600 fully furnished bedrooms. It was too good to pass up.

Seán Dunne's legal team compiled a hefty document that gave me a percentage of the turnover, and specified that I would cover the reopening costs and be reimbursed from the profits within the space of a year. Monthly review meetings would occur to ensure everyone was happy with the progress. I saw no reason to delay and signed the deal which gave me responsibility for their running for a period of one year. Now all I had to do was get them open.

What's In a Name?

had no interest in food and beverage – these were not going to be those kinds of hotels, and the timeframe was too short. And if I'm honest, I didn't want to take on the headache of restaurants and everything that would entail.

I saw these hotels as bed factories: properties that would deliver a good standard of room at a fixed price. Margaret was central to the project and helped me recruit a highly skilled team of 30 people within a week. Patrick Hanley (he of the spelling tests) was on board, as was Michelle O'Donoghue, one of my most trusted colleagues from Kenmare, who would head up reservations and reception.

For this to work we needed a significant web presence, the centre of which was going to be an eye-catching and user-friendly website. And we needed a catchy name. In the bar of the Four Seasons late one Sunday evening Margaret Ryan suggested *D4 Hotels*. It was snappy and memorable, and I thought we could use it to build an online portal for other types of accommodation in the area once the hotels closed for redevelopment when our year was up. I phoned Kenmare and got our General Manager, Rory O'Sullivan, whom I asked to check to see if the name was available on register. com. It was, and he was instructed to buy it immediately.

We had a name, which meant Margaret could get to work putting the marketing side of the project together. As we had three hotels, we needed to bring them all under the D4

Hotels brand. We choose Ballsbridge Inn, Ballsbridge Court and Ballsbridge Towers and registered all the names. Which meant we now had three web addresses under the banner D4Hotels.com.

Thinking Outside the Phone Box

Patrick always thinks outside the box, and has a great eye for unusual styles. While all the bedrooms were furnished, the lobbies of all the hotels were empty apart from carpet and a grand piano. We had no budget, but this did not deter Patrick, who hit on the idea of taking a single chair from each of the bigger bedrooms and with these furnished the lobby overnight. I love that type of thinking: inventive and creative.

The Ballsbridge Court always had a fantastic chandelier in the lobby. It had been removed when the previous owners left, and we needed to replace it with something dramatic. Without any money to spend, I was at a loss. Around the same time Habitat, the homeware store, was closing their Dublin outlet and Patrick went for a look. They had a set of seven oversized lampshades hanging from the roof. Patrick had a chat with the manager and did a deal. He arrived at the store on the Saturday night they closed and bought the shades for €100. We had our replacement. You can't teach problem-solving skills like that, but he is from Kerry so that is his PhD.

When the hotels closed it seems no one thought they would ever reopen. The gas supply pipes were cut off and sealed at the gate, the phone system had been removed with wire-cutters and the lifts were all disassembled. Everything needed to be repaired and set running again, but the phone system offered the greatest challenge. We were planning an internet-based operation and we had no phone line. A single line to create an ethernet connection would have been simple enough, but we needed 30 individual lines and 600 extensions or we would not receive Fáilte Ireland accreditation. Reconnecting such a mess was anything but simple.

On examination I learned the existing wiring was for a Nortel Networking System which is obsolete, and within the time constraints rewiring was not an option. I needed to find out where the Nortel Hub – the machine that permitted the phones to work as an internal network within the hotels and to make calls out – had gone.

According to press reports, the relationship between the previous owners, the Doyle family, and Seán Dunne was acrimonious at best. The Doyles were extremely unhappy the hotels were set to reopen, as they had negotiated first refusal in their sales deal should a new hotel be built on any of the sites, but had overlooked the possibility of anyone reopening the existing hotels. No one in their wildest dreams ever thought they were going to be reopened.

I had a chat with the Doyles, expressing how sympathetic I was to their plight, but explained that I was in a bind, and needed some help. After a long pause they told me they had taken the Nortel system from Jurys with them when they left, as it was to be used as a spare for a similar system in one of their other hotels. The box was apparently being kept in a storeroom in the Westbury Hotel, another property owned by the Doyles.

I was told I could have it for a year, but it was a personal loan to me and if I failed to return when those 12 months were up, I would be liable to an amount of €12,000. The next day I collected the device – a monstrous piece of machinery – and Patrick found two technicians to put it back together. Much to everyone's amazement, it worked. We had lines to all the bedrooms and a connection to the outside world. It felt like the buildings, which had been in a kind of suspended animation, were waking and coming back to life.

Feeding the Troops

Getting food and beverage operators to commit to working with us for a term as short as a year was a difficult task. The effort of building word of mouth and establishing a client base for such a limited time period looked risky at first, but the locations and size were compelling. Within the three properties we had two of the biggest ballrooms in Dublin, the biggest hotel bar, four large restaurants and an equal number of coffee shops ... and I didn't want anything to do with any of them! What I wanted was outlets to service my guests.

I put a package together which I hoped would attract suitable vendors: I wanted no upfront money and no rent; to operate out of one of our Dublin 4 Hotels, the fee would simply be 10 per cent of whatever an outlet turned over. The package must have looked pretty good, because within the space of just a few weeks I had quite a lineup of food and beverage providers lined up to use our hotels as a base of operations: FX Buckley would be looking after our restaurants; Charlie Chawke would be running The Dubliner Bar; Café Java would coordinate the coffee shops and Zumo Juice Bars would provide our more health-conscious guests with a viable option. To complete the package, Blow would be running a line of hairdressing salons and Celtic Cleaners would deal with our laundry and the servicing of the bedrooms on a fixed per-room service fee.

And with that, six weeks after I signed the papers with Seán Dunne, we were open. We were a fully functioning hotel with more than 600 rooms, yet could operate with only 30 staff. It was quite an achievement.

LOW PRICES, NO FRILLS

D4 Hotels offered a fixed room-only rate of €80 per night. There were no supplements for a double or single room – one price fit all. We took out full-page ads in all the daily newspapers, with bold advertising online. We used images of Michael O'Leary saying: 'I don't believe it – low prices with frills!' Another had Carla Bruni saying to her fiancé, the French president Nicolas Sarkozy: 'Ooh La La Nick, look at these rates! We can bring the whole family on the honeymoon.' The ads were cheeky and eye-catching and were intended to get the word out and the phones ringing. They succeeded admirably.

On one day – the day Bruce Springsteen announced he was playing three dates in Dublin – we took more than €150,000 in online reservations. Poor Michelle was run ragged. Most of the booking process was automated, but there was still a lot of filing. Unlike operating in Kerry, where nothing happens but seasonal changes in the weather, Dublin has constant events and massive commercial traffic that flowed to us without any hard graft on our behalf. It is a very different business market. Every concert, conference, meeting, commercial business, national holiday and city break brings business to your door. In Kenmare we have to fight for every room we sell; we don't have all those events that bring business. The scale of Dublin business was an eye opener. All we had to do was keep the costs down, get the word out and the place sold itself.

That's exactly what we did, and within three months we were making tremendously good money. But as we hit the crest of that economic wave the tides were already changing. Ireland was about to enter that recession we've already explored. And the changes came hard and fast.

Our monthly meetings with Seán Dunne and his people turned first into weekly meetings, and before we knew it those weekly meetings were being augmented by hourly phone calls. The plans Seán's team had put in place for the redevelopment did not seem to be working out very well and the banks were under severe pressure and looking for as much money to come in as quickly as possible from every business. Everyone was running for the cover.

Ireland felt like a different planet from the place it had been three months earlier, and on top of trying to deal with D4 Hotels, I had the Park, and The Retreats were just coming to completion.

Seán called a meeting one Thursday evening at 7 p.m. and I had a feeling it was not going to be a cheerful occasion. I said to Margaret we should bring Patrick with us, as it would be a good lesson for him on some aspects of business meetings he had not encountered before. I was right. Seán was not in good form. In fact, he was apoplectic, ranting about costs, returns on investment, incompetent service staff – there was not a single aspect of the project he was satisfied with, and everyone except himself was to blame.

I looked across at Patrick, who was frozen in the seat staring at Seán as if he was a rare breed of predator he had never expected to encounter in the flesh. I, however, was silently smiling, as I knew our time was up and Seán wanted us out, which was okay by me as I had earned my money back at this stage and gained vital experience. In addition, I had no interest in working in such an environment.

I let him rant on for a while, and during a lull where he paused to catch his breath, I said:

'Seán, if you want me out, just say the word and I will walk.'

He leered at me through lidded eyes, before snarling:

'I want you out.'

I smiled warmly around the room, nodded at Margaret and Patrick, and we trooped out. I vacated Jurys, taking the Nortel Phone Hub with me: from the moment I sensed a chill in the air, I had kept wire cutters in the boot of my car, just in case.

Fallout

Margaret, Patrick and I went for a coffee as soon as we left Jurys and tried to decompress and work out what our next step should be.

I already knew though. I phoned our internet provider and instructed them to close the website that handled the bookings. I was well within my rights to do this, as it was ours – my team had designed and paid for it, and they maintained it too, and handled the heavy flow of online traffic that passed through it daily. Of course, without it, Seán's hotels would be unable to continue operating, but that was not my concern.

But I was angry and felt that if me and my people were surplus to requirements, then the skills and resources we had brought to the table must be surplus too. Without the Nortel Hub, and now the website, I had hamstrung the three hotels in a very serious way. And I knew there would be fallout for that. It came quickly. Within 15 minutes of the three of us sitting down I got a call from one of the staff at the hotels to say that all hell had broken loose due to the phone system being disabled, and this was followed shortly by another explosion when it came to light the website had disappeared from the internet. I would have loved to be a fly on the wall when Seán was told; I wish I could say I felt guilty, but that would be a lie.

While working in Dublin I stayed at the Herbert Park Hotel, and that is where I retreated to that night. The moment I got back to my room I wedged the door shut with a chair and prepared for footsteps in the corridor outside, knocks on the door and angry voices demanding I account for my actions. Needless to say, I didn't sleep a wink that night, tossing and turning as I brooded over what had been a punishing period of work, and the anger I knew I had brought down upon myself. As soon as I thought he would be up and about, I called my solicitor.

'I think I'm in trouble,' I admitted.

'You'd better tell me all about it,' was the response, so I did, making sure I left nothing out.

'Okay,' my lawyer said when I was done. 'Here's what you need to do, and you're not going to like it.'

'I'm listening,' I said.

'You need to give them back the phone system and get the website back online.'

'You're right,' I said curtly. 'I don't like that one bit.'

'You've made it impossible for them to continue trading,' he said. 'Let them get back to doing business, and we'll find another course of action.'

I returned the Nortel Hub, but insisted I receive €12,000 in exchange, as the machine was not mine to give, and I would need to pay the Doyles for it. And one phone call sufficed to have the website back online.

I didn't feel good about it, but you do what you have to when you're in the middle of a war. And the fighting was about to get worse. Seán Dunne issued court proceedings against me.

A Day in Court

Seán's main issue was over the ownership of the name *D4Hotels.com* and its accompanying websites. I held that my team had come up with the name, done the branding and developed and maintained the main site and the subsidiaries that applied to the three hotels, but he believed that all intellectual property pertaining to the three hotels was his.

By this time the economy was in the deepest of holes, and there was little material worth in any of this, but I firmly believed in the principle I was fighting for. This was the work of my amazing team. Our ideas, our toil and our passion had gone into creating something special and, regardless of the value of the sites, I was not giving it away.

In the middle of all the turmoil Margaret phoned me a few months later and said the other websites were up for renewal, and what did I want to do. I thought about it for a moment and told her to forget the three sites for the individual hotels, but to keep paying for the domain name, *D4Hotels.com*, as it was the hub and contained the long-term value we had planned for. And I felt D4 Hotels, as an idea, might be a concept I could revisit in the future, if the clouds parted and the economy turned around.

Court cases are miserable things to be stuck in the middle of, but they are never less than fascinating. And this one was *really* fascinating. The case was against me and my company for claiming ownership of the web portal. Unbeknownst to me when I made that phone call to Rory the night we chose the name *D4Hotels.com*, he used the Park Hotel Kenmare credit card to pay for the registration of the domain. Which meant that Seán Dunne was suing me for something I didn't own.

If it hadn't been so serious it would have been quite funny, but then, I always see the funny side of everything, and this did make me laugh quietly to myself. What was even funnier was that, in a document that ran to more than 200 pages, Seán Dunne's legal team never mentioned the term *Intellectual Property Rights*, nor made any reference to the ownership of the name *D4Hotels*. Which played right into my hands.

My solicitors, Gore and Grimes, played a blinder. It soon became clear there was no way Seán Dunne could win, but he had been hog-tied by his own avarice. His legal team had initiated proceedings, so if they pulled out our costs would have to be paid as well as a substantial fee for the web portal. If they continued to do battle it was highly unlikely they could win, as the actual owner of the portal was not even a party to the proceedings, and the contract I had signed did not cover the matter of ownership. It was a perfect example of a group of professionals and legal experts drafting a complex document, thrilled at the dexterity of their wit and guile, but in the process missing the focal point of the thing completely.

I have heard on numerous occasions that the case is referenced in lectures on Law courses as a test case, and so it should be. Which, while a wonderful honour I'm sure, brings with it its own difficulties. Because we were breaking new legal ground, things dragged on even longer than they probably needed to. Costs were astronomical, and every time I thought we were on the verge of turning a corner, another problem raised its head.

Mediation was suggested to avoid us ending up in front of a judge. So far, this was all solicitors' letters flying back and forth, demands for documents and paperwork, fraught meetings and angry phone calls. And every single one of those was billable, meaning it cost me money. Mediation proved a waste of time. Their side was immovable, and so was I. We would have our day in court.

We arrived at the Four Courts loaded down with folders, note pads and the fondly held wish this would soon be over. The court was packed to capacity, as the case had attracted a lot of attention, and the press were very much in evidence. I sat back, and waited for the show to begin.

During Seán's Dunne's testimony I received a tap on the shoulder and turned to see one of his representatives crouched behind me. They wanted to talk. There was much whispering and heated discussion among the lawyers, and I hung back, waiting to see what they would cook up between them. In the end, a settlement was offered, and we took it.

A sum, which I will not divulge here (suffice it to say it was substantial) was to be paid to us, and in return we had to sign over the four domains we had set up and registered to manage bookings and promote the hotels. I refused to leave the court without a signed document, and I also insisted a period of time was set during which money and ownership documents could be exchanged before the case could be officially dismissed. I feared that if we dismissed the case that day, without written assurances and a timeframe for it all to be finalised, we might never get anything.

I was standing on the steps of the courthouse, congratulating myself on our victory when Margaret, ever the pragmatist, reminded me we no longer owned the domains for the three individual hotels: Ballsbridge Inn, Towers and Court. We in fact only owned D4Hotels.com. I almost fainted dead away.

INTERNET INVESTIGATIONS

I had just signed a High Court document I was not in a position to fulfil. If I didn't act quickly, I could be exposed to hundreds of thousands of euros in costs. Without pausing for the dust to settle, I phoned our internet specialist and told him to immediately buy back the three domains. Five minutes later he called and said the Ballsbridge Towers and Court had been secured but *BallsbridgeInn.com* was no longer available. It had, apparently, been bought by a company in Madeira. My blood went cold. Two domains were worthless – we needed all three or the agreement was null and void.

'Find out who has registered it and call me back, even if it's four o'clock in the morning!' I instructed.

My internet detective called me back within five minutes and said a subsidiary of Register.com was behind the action, and would be happy to sell me the domain for €10,000. This, I learned, is a common ploy. Companies like Register.com keep an eye on domains that have high volumes of traffic and, if they aren't renewed they reregister the names with a view to reselling them for a tidy profit. Internet law dictates the price they offer cannot be increased and they must wait a month before selling. Which meant I would need to stall Seán Dunne's legal hounds for a month while the waiting period elapsed.

Meanwhile my internet specialist had decided he was going to save me some money, and suggested we offer €5,000 for the domain.

'Nobody,' he informed me in horrified tone, 'and I mean *nobody* ever pays the full asking price in these situations!'

'I really do appreciate your desire to protect my interests,' I told him, trying to sound grateful rather than like someone who was about to have a cardiac arrest from stress, 'but I am instructing you to get on the phone or to send an email or to compose an instant message or whatever it is you use, and tell those people we will pay them their full asking price, and that they're to get the wheels in motion without delay!'

Muttering ominously about this just not being the way it was supposed to be done, he did as he was asked, and we secured the deal a month later.

I will never forget the joy and relief of being able to return to court and close that case. It was one of the most turbulent experiences I had ever been through, but I still don't regret working on the project. I gained experience I never would have had, and I proved to myself that I could take charge of something vast and multi-faceted and make it happen in a very short space of time. There were countless problems that required my team to think outside the box and make rapid decisions, and we saw all those through with deft assurance. If the recession hadn't delivered a death blow to the economy, things might have ended differently.

To wrap up the story, I'd like to say a few words about Seán Dunne. His vision for those sites was ahead of its time. I must stress that no one achieves the success that man has enjoyed without vision, guts and determination. You may question his methods and disagree with his tactics but behind the fuss and bluster is a trait few have: an iron will to succeed. Seán Dunne and developers like him may have been part of the problem that brought Ireland to its knees, but they also were the people who saw opportunity, grasped it and strived to create something new and dynamic. I learned a lot from working with him, and I never bear a grudge. I hope he feels the same way.

PART TWELVE

Let's Go Glamping

Pitching for Dromquinna

With the D4 Hotels debacle behind me I refocused on
Kenmare. It was my first love and would always
be where I was happiest and felt at ease.

Gwen and I live seven kilometres from Kenmare, and each
day on my way to work I used to pass an estate, Dromquinna
Manor. Built on 40 acres of parkland, it was on a magnificent
waterside setting complete with a boathouse and outhouses.
It had been a hotel back in the eighties but had been bought
by an English company to develop into a kind of smaller
version of a Center Parcs-style attraction. They made an
application to the planning office that had plenty of local
support, but three attempts to secure planning failed, and in
the end they sold up and headed for greener pastures.

I thought it a shame, as the developments they completed
in England, which were around the Lake District, were
first class and trade successfully today. I always feel bad
when a place like Kenmare loses international investment,
too. A local or national investment brings no new business
but dislodges it from another area, whereas international
investment carries all its marketing strength with it and
breathes fresh life into a locality.

With the English investors gone, an Irish consortium
(group of companies) stepped in. I am always nervous of
consortiums, as I think they are purely there for a quick
return and not for the long-term welfare of a business or

a community. They lodged an ambitious plan for a hotel development that would have more than 500 bedrooms along with leisure and conference centres. This carried an estimated development cost of more than €70m – ambitious by any standards, but this was 2004 and the country was awash with money.

Much to everyone's surprise, the Dromquinna application was granted planning, and the way was paved for the redevelopment. For reasons I have never been clear on the consortium folded, however, and the file was left sitting on the shelf of some isolated office of the Allied Irish Bank. Not in liquidation or receivership, but just sitting there. Doing nothing. It was extremely odd, and struck me as a huge waste.

On my daily commute I watched Dromquinna's slow demise. A Limerick security firm was employed to stand watch over the premises. They set up shop in the gate lodge, and I noted they had three rotating shifts. I could not believe a team of security guards was being paid to be in situ while a property effectively crumbled around them from disuse. But that is precisely what was happening.

Years passed. By the time we rang in 2009, Dromquinna was basically derelict. Along with the rest of the country, I was far too busy trying to keep my business from going under to be even vaguely interested in new projects, but I would often pop over to Dromquinna by boat – I arrived via the river to avoid the eyes of the security man who was watching the road entrance – and have a ramble around.

The security detail rarely left the gate lodge, so I was free to wander the grounds and have a good poke about. And everywhere I looked I saw potential. Beleaguered as I was by financial worries on all sides, I tried not to think about what could be done on this land, but my mind kept turning it over anyway. Sheds in the middle of nowhere in County Meath were fetching insane prices, and this superb waterfront estate was all but abandoned. It just didn't make any sense, and in addition no one was asking why or kicking up a fuss. It was as if it had simply been forgotten.

I was pinned to my collar with the Hotel and Retreats, yet with what time I could spare, I began to pursue Dromquinna. Maybe I have a masochistic streak. Or maybe I just hate to see something beautiful being allowed to die. Whatever the reason, the place seemed to be calling to me. And I felt compelled to answer.

ON THE SHELF

B y the time I started looking the trail was already cold. After some subtle investigating I discovered the bank was paying a security firm €300,000 a year to occupy the Gate Lodge of the property and do absolutely nothing else. When I heard this, I was sure I could present the bank with a deal they couldn't refuse – one in which they were *earning* money on the property rather than simply haemorrhaging cash on something that was bringing them no benefit. I just needed an opportunity to talk to the person who dealt with the file.

I phoned a friend in AIB. Could he find out for me who had their property in their portfolio? My friend came back a few days later and said his bank did not have the property. That flummoxed me, as I was convinced AIB had the file. Dad used to tell me that, if at first you don't succeed, go over the person's head, right to the top if you have to. I have always found it good advice, and as luck would have it one of the very senior executives in AIB was a client of the hotel. I phoned him and explained the situation. He called me the following day with the same response: 'We don't have it.' This time I knew how to counter, though.

'Could you do me one last favour?'

'If I can.'

Could you see if you are paying a salary to a security firm

to watch a property just outside Kenmare? Because if you are, then you *do* have this property.'

It took my friend three weeks later to follow the necessary paper trail, but he did finally call me.

'The file was sitting on a shelf in an office, not assigned to anyone,' he told me in tones of wonder. 'It basically has effectively been dormant, and still would be if you hadn't asked about it.'

'Glad to have been of service,' I said.

'We'll assign it and whoever is appointed will contact you in the coming days.'

It had taken me years, literally, but Dromquinna was finally within reach. Almost. It turned out to be months before I received a call from AIB Limerick. Having revised (dusted down) the file, they were going to put the property on the market. I was massively disappointed.

'Couldn't we just sit down and work out a deal?' I asked.

'We have to be seen to be transparent,' was the response. 'The property must go on the open market.'

I hung up and realised that this news presented me with another problem. If someone else bought Dromquinna, I might be faced with the reality of them developing another hotel or guest house within only a few miles of the Park, which could cause untold pressure and put a strain on business we were already struggling to get in through the door in 2010. But there was nothing I could do but wait and see how everything played out.

CBRE (Coldwell, Banker, Richard, Ellis), the world's largest commercial real estate firm, produced a glossy colour brochure on Dromquinna that included maps, photos and a cleverly written blurb that outlined what an amazing opportunity this was for whichever buyer was lucky enough to finally own the property. And the competition was on. It was up to me now to make sure Dromquinna and I were finally united.

My pitch was twofold. The first offer was to lease the property for the full asking price for a period of up to six years by paying a rent equal to the interest on that asking price. While doing that I would undertake to refurbish with a view to reopening and I wanted an option to buy within a six-year period at a fixed price. The offer was backed up with a detailed business plan that made the whole thing more attractive, I hoped.

I told myself the bank would see they would be saving the ludicrous expenses of security, they would get the interest on the price they wanted and if I withdrew at any stage, I would be leaving the property in a much better state than I had found it. The risk to them was that, if my business failed, it might be messy and cause problems down the line. AIB only wanted to close files and bring money in, so it was a big ask.

I knew I was never going to be able to find the capital to open a hotel, and quite frankly, neither the area nor the country, for that matter, needed another hotel. I decided instead to create a luxury camping and wedding destination which was the basis of the Business Plan.

What I was proposing is now called 'glamping' – glamourous camping, or glammed-up camping, if you prefer. It was a brand-new idea back then, although is now extremely popular. There was nothing like it for miles around, and it would give me a chance to explore a new facet of the hospitality industry. Surely anyone would see it was an idea that made sense? I knew, however, that I was dealing with suits wanting to close files, not build business and create employment.

DOING THE DECENT THING

As I told you a while back, the man who developed the Park Hotel and brought Francis in as General Manager was called Mr Weeland, and he had departed Ireland in the late eighties to make a fortune buying and selling property in Dubai.

He had also bought and sold a lot of land in south Kerry, and had an abiding love for the area. By the second decade of the 21st century he was not around as much as in the past, but he came to stay with us from time to time, and on one of those occasions bought an apartment from me at The Retreats.

That night he went to a local restaurant, Mulcahy's, for dinner and I sent a bottle of champagne so he could toast the apartment purchase. Next morning over breakfast he informed me that he had heard Dromquinna was for sale. My heart sank, as he had owned Dromquinna twice in the past and had the means to buy it again if he so wished. I told him I had a bid on the property and outlined what it was. He listened, smiling sweetly, before informing me that, if he chose to buy it, I could rest safely in the knowledge he would not be turning it into a hotel. Later that day he put in a cash bid €100,000 more than mine.

CBRE issued a closing date for bids and there were two of us in it. I was in a two-horse race: in one lane was a cash purchase, in the other a lease risk but perhaps a better outcome for the bank in the long run. I waited, hoping against hope my clearly thought-out pitch would emerge victorious. Weeks passed without news, and then one morning I received a call to say CBRE had just extended the date for final bids – basically an attempt to see if either of us would increase their offer. I resubmitted the exact same pitch, gritted my teeth and continued to wait.

It was coming to the end of shooting for *At Your Service* in that year's season, and Francis and I were filming a campsite in Roscommon. The owners were a lovely couple who had the intelligence, resilience and work ethic to make their business a success; they just needed to be nudged in the right direction.

It was one of those scenarios where we knew we needed a hook, something to hang that episode's story on, and Francis suggested I give them the glamping idea. I was absolutely not in favour of doing so, and I told him it wasn't for public airing as I wanted the idea for Dromquinna. My brother pointed out to me, in his gentle way, that by this stage I had been looking at Dromquinna for three years and the project was stalled. It seemed to be going nowhere. The show needed a story, this lovely family needed a helping hand, and anyway, Roscommon is miles away from Kenmare. We were hardly going to be in competition with one another.

Knowing he was right, I gave in and brought the couple to a glamping location in England, one I had visited in my research. I saw the same range of amazement, inspiration and excitement play across their faces, and I knew they were seeing the possibilities. They went home, and made their site a huge success.

I had mixed emotions. I had given away my idea, handed over one of those elusive USPs, which is something I had vowed never to do. It turned out to be a great show, though.

Think Tanks

One day I got a call from a Dublin-based businessman representing a man called Chuck Feeney, the Irish-American billionaire who made his fortune from creating duty free shopping. His 'boss' was interested in buying Dromquinna Manor and turning it into a kind of residential Davos, where captains of business could come for brainstorming meetings. It was a superb plan that would work well in Dromquinna, would bring a new client profile to Kenmare, and could help create a unique world hub for business leaders. Another win/win.

Whatever hope I had of out-bidding Mr Weeland, I did not have a hope of succeeding against Mr Feeney. At the same time I was heading up a serious project for Kenmare called The Centre of Contemporary Irish Culture (CCIC). We were aware that the Guggenheim in Bilbao had transformed that part of Spain by creating an architectural masterpiece dedicated to the arts, which was drawing one million visitors a year. Ireland had no such facility, as all our main attractions are natural: the Cliffs of Moher, Wild Atlantic Way, the Copper Coast and so forth. Kerry needed a world-class arts attraction to fuel the growing market of experiential and educational tourism.

We had a wonderful committee put together, a stunning plan by Níall McLaughlin, support from all local quarters and eleven million euros raised, which was two million short of making it happen. Pondering how to get Mr Feeney off the scent of Dromquinna, I proposed the following to his Dublin agent:

◊ A full-time think tank centre at Dromquinna would bring an annual cost to Mr Feeney.

◊ I would rent/lease the Park Hotel Kenmare to him for the cost of running it for five months of the year, thus fixing his exposure, a deal that could be terminated at any time with no capital outlay whatsoever. (As the Park was closed for five months anyway I was actually keeping it operational and covering the base cost, so a win-win.)

◊ In return for two million euros we would name the CCIC in his name.

If Mr Feeney accepted, I would get the CCIC built and increase the footfall to Kenmare. I could also keep the team in the Park employed full time and have a good chance of getting Dromquinna. Can you imagine my excitement?

A week after the pitch the phone rang and it was the agent from Dublin. Mr Feeney, he informed me, loved the idea but had lost interest in creating the think-tank centre, so would not be pursuing my proposal. I was disappointed, as it probably meant the end of the CCIC, but it also eliminated a serious contender for Dromquinna. I decided to chalk it up as a win.

PART THIRTEEN

The Big 'C'

Asymptomatic

I did my best to keep a dialogue open with the bank, but weeks turned into months and there was still no news on Dromquinna. Nature abhors a vacuum, however, and during the lull events took a turn that would distract me somewhat from my business dealings. As the wait for word started to become interminable, I began to experience horrendous pains in my stomach. They weren't constant, and days and weeks would pass without any discomfort, but then I'd have a night where I barely slept a wink and where it felt as if my small intestine was trying to escape through my belly button.

Gwen eliminated curries, garlic, and even my beloved wine, but nothing seemed to make a difference. I told myself I was just reaping the rewards of too much good food and tried to force any worries from my head. Whatever it was, it would pass, I thought. Nothing to be concerned about. But there was.

There came a Saturday night when the pain was so bad, I spent the night pacing the floor, sometimes doubled over in paroxysms of agony. On Sunday, exhausted and now convinced I really *did* have cause for concern, I phoned my sister, Catherine (Kate), who works with the President of the Royal College of Surgeons, told her my symptoms, and asked her to recommend the best doctor she knew of. She did, and after that, things moved quickly.

By Tuesday I was in Cork University Hospital, and on Friday I had my gallstones removed by the extraordinarily talented surgeon Morgan McCourt, who operates when not indulging his other passion of surfing. He came to my room after the surgery and told me everything had gone well.

'As we suspected, it was gallstones,' he informed me, 'and I took the gall bladder as well. No need to be alarmed – you won't need it.'

'That's fantastic,' I grinned. 'I take it I can return to curries and wine?'

'All in moderation, but yes, all those treats are back on the table.'

I went home and straight back to work, and I'd never felt better. I was just as full of energy as I had always been, and I greeted each new day and the challenges it brought with vim and vigour. Dromquinna remained frustratingly close while still out of reach, but I had other things to occupy my mind, and I made the decision to focus on those instead and not waste my efforts on a situation I couldn't change.

Two weeks later Morgan called me out of the blue.

'I need to speak to you, John,' he said.

'Alright,' I said, 'well, I have five minutes now, so what's the story?'

'Remember I told you I removed your gall bladder?'

'You said I wouldn't miss it. Are you calling to say you've decided to put it back?'

'No,' the surgeon laughed. 'John, lots of people have nodules on their gall bladders, and most are completely benign. There was quite a large one on the side of yours, though, and when I removed it, I sent a cell sample away for analysis.'

'Okay,' I said. 'I presume you found something you're unhappy about.'

He paused for a moment.

'We found cancer, John.'

I heard the word and I registered it, but what kept running through my mind was that I wasn't sick. I felt perfectly fit and well.

'What does that mean, Morgan?' I wanted to know.

'I want you to speak with a specialist,' he said. 'This is not my area of expertise, so I've made an appointment for you to see Professor Mary Cahill next week. She's the best there is, and she'll look after you.' I agreed to see the professor, and we hung up. I stood where I was in my office in the Park, thinking about what I'd just heard. And no matter how I tried, I couldn't get my head around it.

A Six-Letter Word With a Lot of Baggage

L et me tell my dyslexic friends that cancer has six letters, but is a much bigger word than its size and composition suggests. It carries a weight of expectation and dread, but it is not the medical bogeyman it once was. Medical science has come on in leaps and bounds over the past 20 years, and illnesses that were once death sentences are now conditions people can carry while continuing to live full and contented lives.

Once again I have to state: I was not ill. I'd been told I had cancer, but as far as I was concerned that morning, it might be nothing more serious than a toothache. I wasn't going to get overly upset. Gwen, on the other hand, was a different kettle of fish, and was devastated, but she and I have always been able to talk about things, and together we agreed that, no matter what news I received the following week, we would face it together and support one another in whatever way we needed to. My wife assured me she would be strong for me and for the kids, but we'd been married for a long time, and I knew she was gutted. She did her best to put on a brave face, though, and I loved her for it.

I was filming for *At Your Service* in Tipperary on the morning of 16 March 2011, the day I was to meet Professor Cahill. I finished up the scenes we were capturing, trying to keep my attention on the task at hand and not reveal how rapidly my mind was racing. I must have done a good job, because the director told me he was happy with my efforts, and I hopped in the car and drove to meet Gwen in Cork. We were both extremely nervous as we waited to see the professor. We didn't know what to expect.

The only information I had been given was that some cancerous cells had been found. What kind of cancer these cells were, what the implications of that might be, what impact they could have on my life expectancy, what the possible treatment options were – these and a hundred other questions swam about in our minds.

We met Professor Cahill, who turned out to be one of those people who just ooze competence and calm. She told us I had non-Hodgkin lymphoma, a cancer that is treatable though not curable. I hadn't heard of the disease, as I am not at all medically minded. Gwen, on the other hand, would have a very competent knowledge of the workings of the body, and knew the contents of the next paragraph quite well.

Non-Hodgkin lymphoma is a blood cancer. Symptoms include enlarged lymph nodes, fever, night sweats, weight loss and extreme tiredness. At its most extreme, the sufferer can experience bone pain, chest pain and severe skin irritation. I listened to the professor relating all of this to us thinking that there had to be a mistake, as I never had even the slightest twinge of any of the awful things included on that list.

'Are you sure the files haven't gotten mixed up?' I asked, incredulous.

Gwen shushed me.

'How will you treat it?' she wanted to know.

Professor Cahill said I would have successive courses of chemotherapy, each of which would suppress the effects of the cancer for varying periods of time. There were possible side effects, which included nausea and vomiting, loss of appetite, painful skin rashes and hair loss, but there was no way of knowing if I would experience any or all of them, so I decided to put any worry of that aside and just be glad the prognosis was about as positive as one could expect with a cancer diagnosis.

The cancer was situated in my stomach, and the treatment the professor felt would serve me best as a first course would not cause me to lose my hair, which was good news. Following this raft of therapy she told me it would, with any luck, be five years before I need more treatment, and by then medical science would have evolved and there could be medicines and remedies available we did not even know about yet. So it was all to play for.

We thanked the professor and left, both a little dazed, and I faced a world with cancer a looming new presence.

It Never Rains But …

After leaving Cork University Hospital that day Gwen and I were both numb. Gwen, God love her, had to drive back to Kenmare with a million thoughts running through her head. I headed back to Tipperary to finish filming. My focus was shattered and the last thing I wanted to be doing was filming. But the location was booked, the crew were all on site, and there was nothing to be done but to suck it up and get on with it.

On the way to the location, I phoned Francis to break the news. As I have already discussed, Francis is a deep person, who rarely shows emotion. He took it as well as I expected. And that's as much as I need to say about that.

On the drive to Tipperary I had some dark moments. I am a glass half-full kind of person, but at the end of the day I was facing cancer and chemo, a disease where the cure is almost as horrific to countenance as the illness itself. I like to think I'm strong and see myself as resilient, but I had grown up in a home with a father who was ill, and I knew the impact that had had on my mother and the rest of us. I didn't want to be that father. That husband. And I had to face the possibility I may not have any choice about it.

I reached a fork in the road (not a symbolic one, but I suppose it was that too). One road took me to Tipperary and the film crew. The other would bring me to the Cliffs of

Moher. A long, sheer drop into the ocean. I could end this horror before it began.

It was a momentary flash, nothing more, before I took the turn for Tipp and whatever my life was to bring. But it would be unfair of me to suggest I didn't have that moment. I was back with the crew for 1 p.m. and filming half an hour later. I have never watched that episode and I expect I never will. But I must have looked shell-shocked during my sections. I have always been surprised no one noticed. It makes me think I must always look less together than I have believed.

At 3.16 p.m. that afternoon I received the following email:

16/3/2011 3.16 p.m.
Ref: Dromquinna Manor
Dear Mr Brennan,
We refer to the above matter and to our letter of the 1st of March 2011 and your subsequent letter of the 4th of March 2011 to Paul Collins.
We wish to confirm that our client has considered the proposal and confirm that our client is agreeable to entering a lease with Cloud Nine Services Limited and a Purchase Option Agreement.

For those of you unused to the understated and slightly obtuse language of business, allow me to translate: Dromquinna was ours! I had a moment of elation before reality came crashing in. The morning's news was still fresh in my mind, and I immediately thought: *How the hell am I going to tell Gwen?*

I contemplated the situation for a while and, with a script hastily written in my head, I phoned her. The conversation went as follows:

'Hi! I have some good news and some great news.'

'I'm not sure anything will sound like good news or great news today, but I'll bite,' Gwen said warily. 'What is it?'

'Well, the good news is that the cancer is treatable and not terminal.'

'I was there when we got that bit of news, John. But the other side of that is that it is still cancer. So I fail to see how it rates as *good* news. What's your great news then?'

'Well, the *great* news is,' *(I took a deep breath)* 'that the bank has accepted our offer, and Dromquinna is ours!'

(After a long and ominous pause...) 'Are you serious? I mean, are you out of your mind? We are not doing Dromquinna, John! I don't want a big house with no roof, and you dead from stress and over-work, never mind cancer, leaving me with two kids and a push mower looking at 40 acres of grass ...'

(Having listened for about ten minutes) 'Okay. We'll see.'

Sometimes I don't know if I'm brave or just foolhardy.

Big Brother Knows Best

When I hung up from my cheerful conversation with Gwen I called the bank and asked for documentation to be drawn up.

On a side note, during the call with the bank I asked what swung the deal my way. Apparently the previous Sunday night the episode of *At Your Service* about the campsite in Roscommon – the one where I advised them to try their hand at glamping – was aired. The guys in AIB saw the programme and watching it, understood what my vision was all about. So they decided it was a vision that would work in Dromquinna and they would be willing to take the risk. If we hadn't given the idea to that couple in Roscommon, we may never have got Dromquinna. In my experience, good deeds always foster rewards.

There was nothing more I could do then, so I went on with the day's filming, trying to pretend I wasn't now stretched as thinly as it was possible to be on all fronts. Maybe Gwen was right, and I *had* lost my mind.

That night I had to stay in the guest house where we were filming, and I did not sleep a wink. I remember the room well. It had a pink, outdated sink and bath, and brutal water pressure. There were cream nylon sheets, flower-patterned curtains that would not look out of place in Father Ted's living room, and a worn carpet that was shiny in places from use. But that was not the issue.

My brain would not switch off and let me sleep. My thoughts lurched from how I was going to make Dromquinna a success to worries about a future that might bring with it years of sickness – a life similar to that of my father. I wasn't sure I could endure that with the same dignity he had.

One minute I was as high as a kite, the next drenched in a cold sweat and trembling with dread. It was the worst night of my life – a dark night of the soul if ever there was one, and those curtains didn't help! Morning came, and if I had presented with a white pallor the day before I must have appeared virtually transparent today. Poor Francis was not much better.

The first shoot in the morning was down at the river and Maggi, our director, is not a morning person. All I wanted was to get home, but she couldn't decide on what she wanted to shoot – which angles and backgrounds the scenes called for and where best to capture the light. The debate and discussion and irritating indecision went on and on, and I became more and more agitated. Finally I lost my composure, and with it my temper. Voices were raised, and words were said. Ken, our cameraman, a man who does not enjoy confrontation, zoned out and started looking into the middle distance, always a sign we've crossed a line and need to find our way back over it.

Francis, being Francis, stepped in and, knowing why I was not myself, suggested a perfect selection of shots that would serve ideally. He was just trying to defuse the hostile atmosphere, but it was still too early for Maggi, and his overtures were met with a further lack of decisiveness. Deciding I'd had enough and they'd just have to get through it without me, I departed for Kenmare and the crew went for lunch.

After visiting the Park to make sure all was well, I scaled the wall at Dromquinna and walked the entire 40 acres – the security man appeared to be asleep, again, as no one showed their face and I explored my new acquisition completely unmolested. Maybe I was feeling delicate because of the high emotions of the past few days, but I found the fields, woods and water of the place quite moving. It looked so sad but so full of potential. I knew I could breathe life back into it – I knew I *had* to.

I arranged a group of people whose opinion I respect to come and view the site. Paul Deevy from Richmond House in Cappoquin, Pat Sheahan our accountant and of course Margaret Ryan were to come the following week to have a look at the area and hear what I had in mind.

As we had nothing signed, we pretended Paul was an American investor coming for a viewing with his advisors, and I had just tagged along as he was staying in the Park. It was a glorious day, and we covered the entire property, opening the doors to rooms in the manor that had not seen footfall for over a decade. Everyone was blown away by what they saw. Afterwards we all retired to my house for drinks, where my advisors regaled Gwen with their opinions that there was no negative to be seen in this deal. All it required was guts and hard work. And those were things we had by the boatload. I could tell she was coming round. Slowly.

Rights and Wrongs of Way

The documents were drawn up and were to be signed by the weekend of 31 March. The one issue I was adamant about was rights of way, which is an issue I hate. In rural areas they can be very complex, with thoroughfares crossing land owned by other people, and it all gets very confusing and problematic. It is something I have no patience with. As far as I'm concerned, you either own something or you don't.

I went to the bank's solicitor's house in Cork to sign the deal, as it was after 6 p.m. when I got to Cork. I was assured all rights of way had been terminated, but on looking over the documents there was one in the name of Mrs B_____. It was an unfamiliar name – I knew everyone in the area – but I assumed it must be someone who had lived there years ago and moved away, so I phoned two local people who knew everyone in the Templenoe area for the past five decades. They'd never heard of her.

I was furious and informed the solicitors I would not be signing. I really was livid – to have come all this way, spent years chasing this location, only to have it snatched away at the last hurdle over something so seemingly insignificant was outrageously frustrating. But insignificant or not, I would not commit to millions of euros and years of work, only to have someone come along at some unforeseen point down the line claiming they had a right to come on my land and walk wherever they wanted to at any time. I would rather not sign at all. At that point Francis phoned to see how things were progressing and I told him the news. Quick as lightning he informed me:

'That's Mr Weeland's ex-wife's maiden name.'

I went numb. The man who had owned Dromquinna twice before and had gone up against me in the bidding now seemed to have a right of way through the property. I told the lawyers I was walking away. It broke my heart to do it, but by now you'll be well aware that I hold my principles very dear.

Much to my amazement I got three phone calls that night, from the estate agent, a senior bank official and the bank's solicitor's boss, all pleading with me to reconsider. I laid out the facts to each of them, and they boiled down to one, simple conflict: the deal I had been presented with stated that Dromquinna was right-of-way free, but the title revealed it was not. So there could be no deal.

Next day my solicitor, who happens to be my brother-in-law, Michael Monahan, called me with some very welcome news. On close scrutiny of the maps accompanying the file, the right of way only related to a piece of land on the *other side of the road*, so had no impact on the main estate. He called the bank on my behalf to say I might be prepared to reconsider my position. A small sweetener was added to the document and I signed on Sunday afternoon.

No hotel was sold in Ireland in 2011. Business all over the country was still at a standstill, but my plans for Dromquinna stood out to the jaded officials at the Allied Irish Bank as something fresh and innovative, something they were willing to take a punt on. To their credit it was a brave decision, as all they really wanted was to close the files and wipe bad debt off their books.

It is however a lesson that you don't really need big money in the bank to make things work. Structure your deal to be a win-win and you have a good chance of succeeding. In our wildest dreams, Gwen and I never imagined we would own an estate like Dromquinna, and especially not on that 10-hour journey from Sligo after selling our dream home.

Never have I been so grateful that I allowed Francis to talk me into giving that nice couple my glamping idea, as Dromquinna would not have happened if we didn't. I think it was karma stepping in. A leap of faith and an act of kindness brought me some good luck, just when I needed it most.

Two Veg and Potato

All of that acted as a distraction, but in moments of quiet, the first thing that came to my mind was that I had non-Hodgkin lymphoma. I should not have cancer, I decided, and going for chemo just seemed like a cruel joke. I'd had gallstones, which had been removed, which meant I was now 100 per cent healthy.

'If at first you don't succeed, go over their heads' was wisdom that had stood to me recently, so I was sure it would on this occasion, also. I phoned Professor Paddy Murphy from the Sloan Kettering Cancer Treatment Center in New York. He is one of the leading cancer surgeons in the United States and had stayed with us in Kenmare. I told him my story, sent him my files and got the following reply:

You are with one of the best in the world with Mary Cahill. She might not hear of every advance as quickly as we do here, but if we hear about something today, she will have heard by tomorrow. If I were you, I would stay right where you are.

So that was that.

Tommie Gorman, formerly RTÉ's Northern Ireland journalist, is from Sligo and had christened me 'man child' when he was a regular (if restrained) drinker in Beezies all those years ago. Tommie had his own battle with cancer, and had experienced far more severe symptoms than me. I told him my news and he said in characteristically plain English, as is his skill:

'John, you have two veg and potato cancer. It's straightforward and treatable, and therefore nothing to be afraid of.'

I found this simple, yet profound, and it altered how I thought about my circumstances from that moment onwards. This was a minor setback, but it should in no way alter my plans or make me rethink my life choices. I had two veg and potato cancer, which was mundane, mainstream almost, and therefore not worth agonising over.

I started treatment without telling anyone in the Park or any of the new team in Dromquinna; without informing any of our friends or neighbours in Kenmare; and without bothering my mother with the news. Neither she nor anyone else needed to know. Months passed and no one was any the wiser. I suffered no side effects, my performance as General Manager was unaffected and I was happy in the knowledge I had made the correct decision.

The treatment was delivered intravenously directly into my arm. It took about seven hours for the first load to be delivered, and each subsequent dose was a little shorter – the second five hours, the third four. The best I can say about how it made me feel was that I was fine while I was receiving the therapy, but later that day I'd be hit by severe fatigue, which meant I was utterly exhausted. Then a couple of days later, the steroids would kick in and I'd be high as a kite and couldn't sleep.

But while this was unpleasant, it was manageable. Professor Cahill warned me, though, that the status quo could not remain unaffected.

'You'll get a few years out of this first course of treatment,' she reminded me, 'but the next one will be tougher. You'll probably lose your hair, and you may be nauseous and tired. I'd think about telling the important people in your life before that happens. Give them some time to prepare.'

I knew she was right on an emotional level. And it was good management, to boot. At our end-of-year meeting with the management team of the Park, I told them why I had been missing for three days every month. None of them had suspected – in fact, they thought I was in Dromquinna when I wasn't about the Park, and the team in Dromquinna thought I was in the Park when I wasn't there. Having the two properties had brought me a clear advantage! For all that my team were emotional as I knew they would be, they were also warm, supportive and, most of all, kind. I had no doubt they would be there for me if things got tougher.

I don't want to dwell on my cancer. It is something I have to live with, and it isn't ideal and I wish I didn't have it, but it could be far worse. You would not be reading this if I didn't have cancer, as recovery from my second bout of chemo gave me time to write – there's always a silver lining!

I responded quite well to that first course of chemotherapy, and it was eight years before I needed a second one. That was rougher, and did make me feel nauseous, and I lost my hair. But I recovered, and the hair grew back, and the world didn't shake on its axis.

I was invited to go on *The Late Late Show* to talk about my experience of living with cancer, and Francis and I did the show on 15 May 2020. I was very reluctant to go on, but I did it because the show that week was trying to raise money for Daffodil Day, which is organised by the Irish Cancer Society. Ryan Tubridy, the host of the show, is a friend, and the interview was sensitively done, and as painless as such a thing could be. And I helped raise some money for cancer research, which is always a good thing.

Chasing the Queen

A big news story in 2011 was the visit to Ireland of Queen Elizabeth II. She came in May, but I got wind of her pending arrival a little bit beforehand. There were murmurings, both within the hospitality trade and in the media that a State Visit was planned, and I was not going to pass up that opportunity. I wanted to bring the queen to Kenmare. The problem was, I had no idea how to even go about it. However, I knew someone who did.

David Linley, whose furniture and design skills I had used in The Retreats, is a member of the extended British Royal Family – his official title is Viscount Linley. I have great admiration for him, as he was born into a world where he didn't have to ever work, but he had an interest and a skillset and he makes the most beautiful and artfully designed furnishings. He works very hard at it, too. David Linley is not at the top of his profession because he has royal blood. He is there because he is extremely good at what he does, and his products are sublime. I thought David might have an idea how I could get a letter to whoever was organising the queen's visit, so I arranged to meet him in Christie's in London, where he was Chairman, the next time I was over in England.

'I hear the queen is coming to Ireland,' I said after we'd said our hellos and I'd had a tour of the galleries.

'Who told you that?' he asked, sounding a bit horrified.

'I have it on good authority,' I replied.

'I think it's very unlikely,' he said, but I knew he was only toeing the party line.

'Let's pretend she is, then,' I said. 'How could I get her to come to Kenmare?'

'You can't. Her itinerary will already have been planned. Hypothetically, obviously.'

'Suppose I wanted to try and change that itinerary? It's the 150th anniversary of Queen Victoria's visit, and if Queen Elizabeth were to come to the town, we would love to host her at the Park.'

'Do you have horses at the Park?' David asked. 'Horses are about the only thing she'll change her plans to see.'

'We don't, but that doesn't mean we couldn't arrange for some to be there.'

He considered for a moment and then said, 'I think you're wasting your time, but I can see how it would be a major coup to have Her Majesty among your list of famous patrons.' He scribbled a name and address on a Post-it note and handed it to me. 'This is the name of one of the queen's advisors. I'll tell him to expect to hear from you. Send him a letter stating your case, and who knows? If the queen does decide to visit Ireland, maybe you'll make the cut.'

I was delighted, and Margaret and I composed the best letter imaginable, outlining the merits of our town, the beauty and historic importance of the area, and how we would make the royals so welcome at the Park. And then we waited.

Two weeks almost to the day I posted the letter, I received an envelope with Buckingham Palace's distinctive post mark. Which was very exciting indeed. The letter it contained was the most carefully composed piece of writing I have ever encountered. It was, of course, printed, but my name had been handwritten in a gorgeous, flowing script. The author thanked me for taking the time to write and told me that there were no plans for the queen to visit Ireland at that time (which I knew was a lie, but secrecy was still the order of the day).

'However,' the final paragraph of the letter concluded, 'if she were to make any such plans, I am sure she would receive many letters of the type you were kind enough to send, so each would have to be considered on its own merits.' It took me a couple of minutes to realise, but Buckingham Palace had sent me a very articulate and polite two-fingered salute. I am dyslexic, after all.

My take-away from the whole episode though was that I had been able to infiltrate the queen's inner circle, however unsuccessfully. But I took it as an achievement in itself. And I enjoyed the knowledge I had tipped them off that we knew she was coming!

PART
FOURTEEN

Caring for the Carers

A Very Special Christmas Special

One of the more personal shows we did with *At Your Service* was a makeover Christmas Special in North County Dublin for a charity called CASA – the Caring and Sharing Association. The charity supports people with disabilities by providing respite care and a social outlet, and while we were obviously in favour of what they do, we had no history with CASA whatsoever.

We both approached it as a circumstance where we were just making a TV show for the sake of making a TV show – yes, it was a good cause, but there are loads of those out there. CASA was selected as a result of a letter written to RTÉ by Conor Dillon from Swords, suggesting the organisation might be the subject of one of our shows. Claire Small, our producer at the time, went for a look and to meet Conor. She phoned me within minutes.

'John, I've just visited the location of our next Christmas Special.'

I was in the middle of something or other in my day job, but I like Claire, so I tried to sound interested. 'That's marvellous,' I said. 'If Christmas weren't six months away I'd be jumping for joy.'

Claire's jovial mood was not to be dampened, however. She was totally captivated with Conor and his story.

She didn't get a much better reaction from Francis, but

neither of us was opposed to the location, so we gave it a thumbs up and went to meet CASA's management team and some of the service users. And within the space of five minutes everything changed. A relationship with CASA that endures to this day was established, and a friendship I deeply treasure was formed.

Telling the Story

The Christmas Special is a 60-minute show as opposed to our usual half-hour format, so in it we have much more potential to tell a detailed story. And CASA offered us plenty of fodder for storytelling. They had a public restaurant, a respite house, a charity shop in Dublin City; then they had Conor himself. And that last item on the list is crucially important. The first three are fantastic in and of themselves and a superb show would have resulted, but Conor brought an intangible ingredient, a dynamic we hadn't expected. And he made the Special really special.

Most of us drift through life, independent, free and unaware of how blessed we truly are. Most of us do what we want when we want to do it. I've had my problems with dyslexia and I've had my personal run-in with cancer, but I am painfully aware that any of the obstacles I have had to face in my life are trivial when compared to those confronted and overcome by someone like Conor.

Circumstances have determined that Conor cannot have the full independence most of us take for granted, but he has an intelligence and attitude brighter than most people I have met, and the force of his personality stops you dead in your tracks.

Conor is a remarkable person, and we knew he was going to be the central thread of the Christmas show.

CHARITY SHOP MAKEOVER

An important element of the fundraising side of the charity was Tried and Tested, a second-hand clothes shop in Phibsboro, North Dublin. When I visited the place I found it very higgledy-piggledy, but it made good money and had a great manager. People would drop in unwanted clothes, which were sorted in a back room and either displayed or sent to one of their other shops, as some items were more suitable for different areas of the city which had a demographic of customer more likely to buy them (different ethnic wear, for example). While the charity had many shops around the country we concentrated on Phibsboro, as it was close to the restaurant, the respite home and Conor's homeplace.

Retail is very different from our business, so to help us with this element of the show we brought in John Redmond, the Creative Director of Brown Thomas. He instantly suggested a total revamp of the interior of the shop and the way the items were displayed. These may seem like little things, but they make an enormous difference to the customers' experience, and are designed to entice them into buying. Shops only survive if you are tempted to spend your money in them. Such retail seduction is a very fine art, and John explained that all the senses must be stirred to make it happen.

With this in mind, the amount of items on display was halved and a new shelving and display plan devised so customers could see a hat on a top shelf, a matching coat or dress hanging beneath with a pair of shoes prominently placed on a bottom shelf. It all made perfect sense, but it takes a professional to add a half shelf or hook so you can insert a belt or a pair of sunglasses for that final master stroke that gets a customer to part with their money.

CASA called on all its supporters to help renovate the store accordingly and a colossal amount of voluntary hours was invested by an army of good-natured people to bring John's vision to life. The result is that the shop continues to be a resounding success. It became a *store* as opposed to a second-hand bric-a-brac outlet. Prices increased and consequently, spend-per-person increased. Which resulted in more resources for the charity, which is exactly what it was all about. The restaurant was another story altogether.

How to Break Bad News

The main problem we faced in dealing with the restaurant was that the people who ran it absolutely loved being involved with it and with CASA. People gave their time to running it on a voluntary basis, and many were quite passionate about what they were doing and genuinely interested in working with food.

In reality though, Ten Fourteen, as the restaurant was called, was costing the charity money. We knew from the moment we walked through the front door that it was never going to make money and would, in fact, always be a thorn in the side of the organisation. This was not an easy truth to tell, however, because so many people were involved, and there was such a lot of enthusiasm and goodwill on display.

I remember another show we did where a lovely couple opened a tea rooms in the wrong location. The couple had no past experience in the business but had bought a pub and the tea rooms was a side project in a house they owned up the road. They had done a good job fitting the place out and the menu and style of the place was faultless. Everything was right *except the location.*

It was 100 metres distant from where it should be and as a result lost money every single day. In the section of the show where Francis and I tell the couple what we think they should do, I was very clear.

'Lose the tea rooms today,' I said. You can't get much more plain or direct than that.

It was a heart-stopping moment (and of course the perfect point at which to cut to a commercial break). The couple were stunned, and not a little heartbroken. You would think I had stabbed them in the back. And I couldn't work out why – the writing was surely on the wall, as that wing of the business was haemorrhaging money, and we had already told them most of the components they were bringing to bear on it were right.

When the camera stopped rolling, they told me they had put the last of their money into the tea rooms, but not only that, they had also invested their daughter's savings in a bid to give her some business experience – the girl was just 14. In truth, they added, it was a last-ditch attempt to make money too, as the pub was running at a loss as well.

And this is an aspect of a show like *At Your Service* that most people don't realise: there are always human stories behind each of the businesses. Francis and I walk away at the end of the shoot, but the owners of the week have to continue to live with the decisions they make, for better or worse.

I was gutted as we awaited their daughter's arrival from school. The tea rooms were her pride and joy, and here I was, only there a few hours and having already rubbished the family's long-term plans and the daughter's first foray into business. I will never forget how I felt – it was just horrible. The poor girl bounced in off the bus full of beans, only to be met with gloom and despair. I knew it was the right thing to do, as the business was never going to work, but very raw emotions, not to mention a child's excitement and optimism, were all in the mix.

Returning to CASA, Ten Fourteen was similar, but the cost base and investment profile were very different. This was in a location with great passing trade and was well fitted with a state-of-the-art kitchen and a nicely appointed dining room, so I thought it might be saved.

We revamped menus, some of the décor and put together a number of fresh marketing initiatives, to conclude with a high-profile relaunch. I did my best, but the show proved that first impressions and gut instinct are usually right. Despite a trojan effort, the restaurant closed shortly after. You can't win them all.

REAL HEROES

While Francis and I were trying to address the needs of these satellite operations, we were painfully aware that CASA had a charity to run: a charity that provided a very important service to a very worthwhile group of people.

Everything CASA does is about giving the carers of those living with disabilities – particularly those with mobility issues – time off while their loved ones are on 'holiday' at the CASA home in Malahide. The time spent there gives the carers their only break from the unremitting task of caring for a family member at home. Most of us who are not faced with that reality are blind to the impact of having to care for a loved one 24 hours a day with little or no support or assistance. It is intense and it is draining.

During the making of the show, I spoke to a parent who never got a full night's sleep. Ever. CASA provides that mother with her only break, and the five or six days a year they look after her child is the only time she gets to live and sleep without worry. It is a holiday for her child, but it is a lifeline for her.

The CASA respite house is a typical detached house, adapted to cater for wheelchairs and a range of mobility challenges. It was funded by donation and an endless list of volunteers who carried out the bulk of the labour. And it needed a lot of work.

The *At Your Service* Christmas Special has the reach to call on businesses and skilled tradespeople, so it can, potentially, make a very real difference. A single mention on Ryan Tubridy or Pat Kenny's radio shows and we are inundated with offers of help.

Windows, doors, gutters, kitchens, furniture, beds, tables, chairs, electrical appliances, toys and medical equipment are all made available, and professional painters, builders, carpenters, electricians, plumbers and gardeners line up to help, usually followed by queues of volunteers offering to do whatever they can.

I have always thought there should be a second crew filming the organisation and management of the project behind the scenes, because that is a story in itself. The show we did on CASA has probably received the greatest reaction of all the programmes we have done, and Conor was its star. He and I remain close friends, and he is as bright as ever, constantly coming up with ideas for businesses, always looking for an opportunity, and never without a smile and a kind word for everyone he meets. Despite the profound physical challenges he faces, being wheelchair bound and dependent on others for many things (his parents need to move him five times each night to facilitate his circulation) I have never seen him downhearted, and he is constantly thinking of others. When we wrapped filming of the Christmas Special, Conor said a few words and thanked each and every person involved without ever having to look at a cue-card – he had every single name off the top of his head.

Now that I think about it, he should write a book. I'd have a word with him about it, but something tells me he's come up with the idea already!

PART FIFTEEN

Messing About in Boats

Almost Losing Dory

I am not sure where the interest came from, but from a very young age I have loved boats. I first went boating when I was 13 years old. We had just moved to Sligo. My sister owned a Dory 14 with a Johnson 60 horsepower engine on the back. I was asked to keep an eye on it, which I did by taking it out on Lough Gill, just down the road from where we lived in Aughamore.

My taking the boat out on a lake was not what my family had in mind, but no one had thought to specifically explain the parameters of how I was supposed to be looking after it, and a Dory is a very safe boat, wide and very solid. Perfect for beginners, which is just as well. I'd been watching the Dory for a few days when one of my best friends, Peter Devaney, called over. I brought him down to the lake to show him the vessel I was by now thinking of as 'mine', and between us we decided to take it for out for a spin.

I don't remember feeling nervous at all, just excited as we launched the boat and pulled the cord. The grumpy Johnson motor spluttered into life and Peter and I took off for the middle of the lake. As we moved out into the expanse of water the boat started to get slower. It was not a fast boat by any standards, so such a deceleration was very noticeable.

After a few minutes there was a wash of water around our feet and we saw that the boat was filling with water – rarely a good sign. We managed to turn her about and Peter started bailing out water with his shoe, as we had neither a bucket nor a bottle. I remember we were in grim silence, both of us knowing the situation was dire: we had no radio, life jackets or buoyancy aids. We didn't even have fenders that we could hold on to should the boat totally sink. We just made it back to dock and, shaking with relief, manoeuvred the boat back on the rusty trailer. It was a massively important lesson. Never go to sea without checking the boat, ensuring you have adequate fuel, have life jackets for everyone, have a working VHF radio and nowadays a mobile phone as well.

When we had the boat out of the water I realised we never put the bung in the hull. This is a small little nut or washer that is removed to let water out of the hull when the boat is on its trailer, and not fitting it when we went out resulted in the boat filling with water. It was another rookie mistake I have never made again. My first trip out on a boat was an unmitigated disaster. But that did not deter me one bit.

MY PATCH OF WATER

Moving to Kenmare brought me closer to the water. The town is at the top of Kenmare Bay, or Kenmare River as it is named on all maps. In the 1600s Cromwell employed a man called Sir William Petty to map Ireland. As part of his remuneration, he was given a large parcel of land, at the centre of which Kenmare lies. As he mapped the countryside he named the bay north of Kenmare as Tralee Bay and the one to the south Bantry Bay, but the bay at Kenmare he chose to call a river. This was because in those days if you owned land that adjoined a river, you had the fishing rights, but that didn't apply if your land adjoined a bay. Sir William was a shrewd operator, that's for sure.

Kenmare River/Kenmare Bay (it's actually the Atlantic, if you really want to get picky about it) is at the top of a 35-mile-long waterway, the width of which is in places 16 kilometres, while in others only 500 metres. It is tidal, salty and majestic. The coastline in this part of Ireland is rocky and wooded, dotted with islands, and every time you look back at the land you are struck by the backdrop of the Caha Mountains and the Macgillycuddy's Reeks. To say it is stunning is a gross understatement.

In the past, large boats departed from here carrying lumber for England. Over the years Kenmare Pier has silted up to an extent that only motorboats and sailboats can access the pier at high tide. As a result, the bay sees little boating, which is a dreadful shame.

I have, at this stage in my life, boated all over the world. I have explored the waterways of the UK and many in Europe. I have navigated waters in the United States and crested waves in the Middle East. Yet I never tire of putting out in my adopted home of Kerry.

This, for me, is a special place, and I get the same thrill out of it now as I did that first day Peter and I nearly drowned ourselves in the Dory.

Holiday Excursions

Whenever we were on holidays we would inevitably rent a boat and cruise a bit of the coast around where we were based. In Cyprus one year, with sun beaming and glistening off the water, we took off with our friends Damien and Angela, plastered in lotion, the warm wind whipping our hair back. Angela would at best be nervous of boats but with me at the helm may be even more scared of what might happen. As we rounded a rocky headland we noticed small fish jumping in the near distance. There wasn't a ripple on the surface apart from those fish.

As we got closer we heard what sounded like a machine gun coming from the land. I remember thinking I had to be mistaken, but it turned out it was indeed a machine gun, and those fish we saw jumping were not fish at all, but bullets from the automatic weapon fire thudding into the ocean.

We had crossed onto the Turkish side of the island and they were firing warning shots to turn us back. And turn back we most certainly did. No one mentioned the fact we'd had such a near miss for the rest of the holiday. That was far from the end of our holiday boating, but I do not think Angela has since entered a boat with me.

The next time we went boating was in West Palm Beach in Florida. We had the use of a friend's house for a fortnight, and nothing would do me but to get on the water. The Intercoastal Waterway is a strip of water that runs through the islands all along the east coast of Florida. It is shadowed by some of the most impressive and stylish yet also hideous and gaudy houses you will ever see. From the road you can only see gates, high walls and hedges, but from the water you can view them in all their awful splendour.

Desperate to get on the water and investigate these delights, I made enquiries and rented a 33-foot cigarette boat, which is a long boat, narrow and fast. We got the keys and were instructed to stay within the markers, as there were sand banks everywhere.

It was a glorious day and we headed south to see a house the Kennedy family owned. As we moved through the water I realised we were surrounded by some of the most magnificent sailing boats I have ever seen: Perini Navis, the most celebrated of sailing ships, were dotted everywhere; there were also Vitters, Alloys and too many more to mention. My eyes were out on sticks – I was in sailing heaven.

Our friends Peter and Cass had come on holiday with us and he was piloting the boat while I was busy looking at houses. With so much to see I felt he was going far too slow and also in the wrong direction, so I took the wheel and pushed the throttle forward.

Bang.

The boat stopped dead and we were thrown forward with surprising force. I staggered up and saw the water around us was roiling and black. My crew of Gwen and Cass were crying and I was numb, sure I had somehow blown the engine. At that moment a big white motorboat came around the corner and its driver shouted:

'You guys have run aground on a sand bank!'

I heard what I was being told, but the information didn't compute. How could we be on a sand bank when we were surrounded by sailing boats with keels as much as 20 feet in the water? Our boat's keel could only be three feet at most. It just wasn't possible.

Peter started to laugh, as he had been driving to the next marker, which I hadn't seen, when I took it upon myself to take the wheel. Unaware of what I was doing, I had driven us onto a sand bank. When the water had settled we could see the bank upon which our vessel was now stranded. The pilot of the motorboat said he could call for help to pull us off.

Twenty minutes later a big red tugboat appeared, a vessel so large and powerful it would not have looked out of place in the North Sea. On the bow they had a harpoon-type gun from which they fired a rope towards us – which landed about five feet short of the boat. The blond surfer dude who was operating the harpoon shouted:

'One of you will have to get that!'

Peter gave me a look that said: You got us into this, so you can get that rope!

I stripped off and, hoping to save some face, leapt enthusiastically off our boat and into the water. It never occurred to me for one moment that the water wasn't deep. I dived in like I had seen Johnny Weissmuller do in the old Tarzan movies. Which was my second big mistake of the day, as the water was less than two feet deep, and I almost knocked myself out.

Everyone on my own stranded vessel, and the sun-kissed Adonises on the tugboat, laughed hysterically as I walked stiffly over and tied the rope to the front of the boat. Within seconds we were tied alongside the tug and the blond surfer dude started calculating.

'Thirty-three feet by $10 plus $200 of a callout fee ... make it $500 and we'll call it a deal.'

I looked at him aghast. This had to be a joke. I was about to say something when I spotted Peter counting out $500 from a wad of notes. I was furious. Blondie, the dude (and he was a real dude) on the rescue boat, would have taken $100 but Peter, who has a similar rescue business for cars, had it paid before I could open my mouth. I don't talk when I'm annoyed, so we continued our trip in silence.

I had seen a restaurant called The Waterside Inn a few days earlier and thought it looked nice. It was about 10 miles up the waterway and we had planned lunch there for two that afternoon. As we approached their marina I spotted a pontoon was available. The marina was full of day cruisers, all glinting with polished stainless steel. The restaurant tables were on a terrace just by the pontoon, dressed beautifully in pristine white cloths. A jazz band played in the corner. It was a classy-looking establishment and we were all starving.

There wasn't a ripple of wind as we pulled up to the marina, and everyone in the restaurant was watching as we arrived. I lined the boat up perfectly and entered the pontoon with expert precision. Peter was on the bow with the line and everything was going perfectly to plan. I was so proud. All the onlookers, most of whom had arrived by boat, would have looked upon our arrival and deemed us expert boaters. Peter put up his hand to indicate I should stop, and he jumped off to tie the line.

Delighted with my performance and thinking the ignominy of that morning's grounding was behind me, I decided to lock the wheel and give the throttles a quick burst of power to tuck in the stern, which was not quite alongside the pontoon fully. In my hurry I turned the wheel the wrong way, and when I pushed the throttles forward the bow of the boat jammed under the restaurant terrace, and every table in the place rocked and shook. Within a split second we went from seasoned mariners to a complete joke. I didn't have lunch but the girls tell me it was lovely. These are the joys of boating.

They say the world is full of two types of boaters: the ones who have run aground and the ones who have not yet. Boating is a perpetual learning curve; much like business.

Buying Boats

Of course, if you want to boat seriously, you can't keep renting. You need to own a boat. So as soon as I could afford it, I embarked on an educational exercise to see what the right boat would be for me and my family.

At this stage in my life my son, Adam, was three and my daughter, Ruth, had just been born, so it needed to be enclosed and have a toilet, a fact that immediately eliminated a vast number of possibilities, as it meant whichever model I was going to purchase had to have a cabin.

I spotted a 26-foot hard-top cabin cruiser for sale in Wexford, which had been built by a Finnish company named Aquador, who build their boats in Cork. The Baltic Sea, which is the area this company build most of their vessels for, is actually very like Kenmare Bay. As Kenmare is technically 56 kilometres inland and the waterway can get narrow at times, the boat requirements for both areas are similar, as Finland has a lot of canals too.

The cabin cruiser, which I duly purchased, served me well, but I finally sold it and bought a 7.5-metre Avon Rib, which was perfect for navigating the waterways and islands about Scotland, something I was keen to do. I loved that boat but it drank fuel, so I decided to buy another one from a company in Antrim called Redbay.

On that boat – which is open, by the way, so you need to have all the wet weather gear on you before taking a trip – Adam and myself have been all around Ireland and Scotland and had the best of times. On a Sunday if I can escape the four of us head for Kilmakilloge and Helen's Bar for a Bulmers and fresh crab on brown bread. It's one of the things I so dearly love about boating – you are making memories all the time. There's nothing quite like it.

With Dromquinna located on the seafront and people's desire to get out on the water I knew we needed something bigger. We ordered an 11.5-metre cabin rib to offer people a toilet, which is always a good idea!

There weren't great omens though, the day Adam and I went to pick it up. We set off into the Irish Sea from just north of Belfast to bring the boat home, and almost as soon as we hit the open water a Force 6 gale blew up. Before long, it had reached Force 8 and we were hammered. We tried to get into Carrickfergus to find shelter, but it was too rough. We continued fighting our way onwards, and tried to set in at Warrenpoint, but yet again the elements would not allow us entry – we would have been torn apart.

I was (secretly) terrified by now, but Adam was having the time of his life. So I figured that if he thought this was all going to be fine, I should probably just relax and make the best of it. Realising it was fruitless to keep going, we turned the boat around and limped our way back to Bangor. It was an inauspicious maiden voyage, but that boat has brought me and my family so much pleasure, I forgave that difficult first experience.

WHY BOATS?

I love boats for the same reason I love motorbikes. It's all about the freedom. I spend my days surrounded by people and anchored to buildings, structures and the land they are built upon. My world is one of order and routine and my job involves constant attention to detail. On any given day I will have to conduct innumerable conversations with countless people, and I must be informed about whatever it is I am talking to them about and have facts and figures at my fingertips.

Each day I go to work I am thinking about the many things that will consume my time before I am even out of bed, and I will still be problem solving and sorting through details when I get back into bed at the other end. Boating removes all of that. When I set aside a day or a weekend or a week (if I'm lucky) for boating, that is all I am focused on. On those days there is just me, the beautiful machine I am piloting, the water and the sky.

I need to know about tides and rock formations and wind speed, but those are all just another aspect of this remarkable pastime. And none of them is stressful. None make any demands.

Gwen often tells me she finds certain aspects of boating an annoyance, particularly the fact that boats – all boats – are notorious for having mechanical difficulties. There is always some small thing or other going wrong with them, and rarely a single trip passes without my having to reach for the toolbox. I can spend whole days on the pier at Dromquinna tinkering about with an engine part or taking apart a piece of machinery that has been giving me problems.

Gwen tells me I don't know how to relax, that I can't switch off. But I don't see that as work or a chore. I'm having the time of my life. Boats, to me, are all about family time, exploration, experiences and adventure. They are simply magical, and bring you to places not many people get to see. Boats are one of the things that make life worth living for me.

PART SIXTEEN

Coming Full Circle

New Endeavours in a Brave New World

The COVID-19 pandemic of 2020 took the world as much by surprise as the economic crash 12 years earlier did. The virus ripped its way across the globe, and as it came, country after country initiated lockdowns – movement and travel were restricted, gatherings had to be curtailed and some countries even had curfews.

It would be unfair to say the entire economy was shut down, as supermarkets and chemists remained open and many restaurants switched to offering a take-away service so they could keep trading, albeit in a very different way than before. But hospitality was one of the industries worst hit. I am writing this book during the second hard lockdown in Ireland, and I am not exaggerating when I say that many smaller operators will not come back when the restrictions are lifted.

Dromquinna has many strings to its bow, but when the first lockdown was enforced we didn't know how long it would last, and we needed to do something to keep the core team employed. In typical Kerry fashion, many of the team have multiple skills and can turn their hand to anything and do it well. I had toyed with renovating an old house on the estate but could never find the time. Our General Manager, James Doyle, is not a person who would enjoy a lockdown and having too much time on his hands. After a brief discussion we decided to embark on attacking the house and turning it into a six-bedroomed house with six ensuite bathrooms so James, Pat and Shane (Dromquinna's hard-working maintenance men) went to work. No lockdown for that bubble.

I could not understand the business model of offering take-away services, as it was labour intensive and packaging was costly. In addition, we do not have the local population to make it profitable or even cover its costs. Early one morning as I lay awake at 4 a.m. – always a good time for ideas – I thought we should produce tubs of precooked food and retail them through local shops. It was a simple idea but one that would keep Benny our chef in work and keep our name out there. At 8 a.m. I went to see Andrea Whyte of our local Centra, who gave the idea 100 per cent support. The following Thursday we made our first delivery and today they are available in many shops from Kenmare to Skibbereen. It is a small idea that has proved fortunate on many fronts.

At the Park we were lucky though. Due to the nature of tourism in this part of Ireland, the Park Hotel Kenmare had always closed for five months of the year up until 2004, so when that first lockdown occurred in March of 2020, we were concerned, but optimistic. I sat a very worried staff team down that March and had a long talk with them.

'Here's what's going to happen,' I informed my crew. 'We will close as directed and avail of all the generous supports put in place, but we will also be the first to open and everyone in this room will have their job back and there will be no pay cuts.'

Nobody complained. When we were permitted to open that summer, all businesses earned enough money in three months to cover us comfortably for the rest of the year. And my team made that happen. I have never been so proud of them.

At the end of the 2020 season, I knew the world had changed and was going to take some time to rebound. I also knew hospitality and tourism was going to have to change. Discerning clients would look for different things to interest them closer to home, as everyone will travel less, for a few years, at least.

I had already noticed that our guest profile has gradually been transforming – a younger and younger demographic was visiting us, and post-COVID I strongly believe that trend will continue, particularly as older people may well be afraid to travel for some time. Just as in the beginning of the noughties the Park needed the spa to remain competitive and relevant, I knew we needed to change again, while protecting the character and essence that make us who we are.

So, while the hotel was closed during the first hard lockdown of 2020, I began a restoration programme. When the doors opened for guests in the summer of 2021, it was to reveal a rejuvenated, modern, crisp and elegant interior, complete with a state-of-the-art kitchen where our talented chefs prepared the most amazing food.

During the renovation process my team in the Park have, yet again, showed themselves to be true professionals and dear friends. I saw chefs lugging about furniture, waiters removing wallpaper and my General Manager scraping old plaster off the ceiling. And they all threw themselves into these jobs with smiles on their faces. John Moriarty, who has been with the Park for more than 30 years, worked seven days a week doing all sorts of things way beyond expectations. Because each and every one of them is wholly committed to the vision my big brother had for this incredible hotel back in the 1980s, they want that vision and dream to continue. The Park opened, fully prepared to meet the public, with an exciting new look and experience but one instilled in the history and reputation the Park has always been known for.

And our guests love it. The style walks a fine line between the Park's trademark olde worlde glamour with modern, fresh, clean design. We were able to offer something new, while never alienating any of our regular clients. It was a resounding success.

During the pandemic, another exciting opportunity presented itself. The Lansdowne Arms Hotel is a small hotel that has been a central part of Kenmare for many years, providing a great service to guests looking for a comfortable and casual experience in the town. I had attempted to buy it on a couple of occasions over the years, but for one reason or another the deal never really happened. However, it went into receivership, and I made an offer to the receiver.

My reason for buying yet another property, particularly at a time when the economy is so uncertain, is very simple. The hotel is situated right across the road from the gate to the Park, and I always worried that, if it were bought by someone with a bit of vision and a flair for development, that little hotel could present us with some serious competition. Alternatively, if it was bought by a person without a vision or interest in the wellbeing of Kenmare, it would be a disaster for everyone. The Lansdowne sits at the top of Main Street, in full view of everyone who comes to the town. It is a showcase property that represents Kenmare in a way no other property has the potential to.

Owning it would add yet another string to our bow. We could draw in a discerning younger client group, and with Dromquinna hosting weddings and functions, we would have a steady stream of customers to direct there during the height of the season.

While I was certain buying the Lansdowne was a good idea, I wasn't sure how Francis would take it. Francis was meeting his accountant, Pat, and they asked me to call in for a moment as there was something they needed clarified. At the end of the chat I said I had put in a bid for the Lansdowne as it had gone into receivership. Pat smiled as he could see the potential, but Francis just looked at me. I am not sure what he was thinking, but I suspect he was wondering how I had the time to think of it let alone do it as I had just completed chemo, was leading a major refurbishment of the Park, Dromquinna had just cancelled over 60 weddings due to the pandemic, every hotel in the country was closed and no planes were flying. There was so much happening; why would I bring more on myself? After Pat asked a few questions Francis, who had been listening intently said:

'You're right. It'll be great.' That was all the encouragement I needed.

While the world was closed, it was easy to see our lives as a little slower and a little smaller. But I never looked at it like that. I saw the lull as a time to build potential. To develop and regroup. To prepare for a relaunch and get in as good a shape as I could for reopening. It was a time of hope and looking to tomorrow.

And that approach worked. Our relaunch was a huge success, and I have never been prouder of my team.

Remember what I said about success: it's all about seeing opportunities and grabbing them with both hands. The Lansdowne is one such opportunity. When the deal was closed I went to see it for the first time. Some things you know are right so there was no point looking at it before we bought it as it was well run, had a good reputation and was there since 1790 so was hardly going to fall down tomorrow. I didn't even get an engineer to look at it as they will only find problems and given the building's age there were of course going to be problems so why pay fees to find out the inevitable? Bottom line was it made sense on many fronts.

When I went in with the team from the Park on that first visit I was dumbfounded. Some hotels and buildings have a happy atmosphere and the Lansdowne has it in buckets. Unlike new buildings, heritage buildings have a personality of their own – a feeling, a warmth, a sense of history you cannot build from scratch. We all just looked at each other and I could sense the excitement about what we were going to create.

FINAL THOUGHTS: IT'S NOT ALWAYS ABOUT THE MONEY

Every time I drive into Dromquinna, I am amazed that I own it. It is the most beautiful place, just spectacular, and I never fail to experience a wave of impostor syndrome – a feeling that someone like me isn't supposed to own a property like this. And when I bought it – by now you know all about that deal – I didn't have a penny. As we started to renovate and develop the property, I had to do a lot of the work myself – I cut back gorse, I (very badly) ploughed some of the fields to create gardens so we could plant vegetables to service the Park's kitchens, and I even helped clean the pond. As I did all of that, I was also deciding what business and markets we were going to target. The fact I didn't have the funds ready and available did not stop me pursuing the property. I knew it was the right thing to do, and I went for it.

Francis did the same thing when he bought the Park. He was a young man with barely any money in the bank, but when he was given the opportunity to buy the hotel he lived and breathed for, he knew he had to jump at that chance. The arrangement he made was very similar – in fact was my inspiration – to the one I made at Dromquinna: the sellers effectively funded the sale, allowing him to lease at a very competitive rate, with a view to him purchasing when he was in a position to do so. Which he did within a remarkably short space of time. Once again, not having the cash to hand did not prevent him from following his dreams. Money is not everything. Mental attitude, however, is. I firmly believe that if you think you are finished, then you are finished, literally. If you think you can make something great happen, then you probably can.

There have been so many times during my journey when all the signs told me the game was over and disaster was just around the corner, but I refused to yield, and instead cast about for opportunities, no matter how slim or far-fetched they may have seemed, and kept on fighting.

In this book I have only had the space to tell you about some of the projects I've been involved in, to give you a taste of what I do. I've done things I never would have dreamed possible as a kid sitting in the back of the class in CUS, scoring in the bottom 10 per cent of the group, barely able to make my way through a single page of any of the textbooks in my bag.

I was lucky to have parents who had faith in me. Siblings who reached out when I needed a hand up. Friends who were always willing to share an adventure. A wife who supported and loved me, even when things got tough and illness and financial ruin seemed to spell doom. I also have a group of the most amazing people working with me – I'm not going to say *for* me, because the truth is they share the dream. Without the staff in all the businesses being so loyal and skilled, nothing I do would be possible.

I know many of you are reading this because you have seen me on TV, and I am grateful for the reach *At Your Service* has given me. We still do it with the intention of helping people, in the hopes the owners we meet and hopefully someone watching at home will get an idea that turns their lives and their businesses around.

The main reason I sat down to write this book also had nothing to do with money. It was all about another very important resource: education. I was very lucky that my parents, in particular my mother, understood that the classroom was not for me. She allowed me to give up school in the middle of my exams for a job on a fruit and veg truck at just 15 years of age. The ups and downs and vagaries of my life after that must have given her loads of grey hairs, but she never once told me I had made the wrong choice.

Somehow, she instinctively knew that I learned by *doing*. I needed to get out and see and experience things for myself, and that is how I teach and train my own staff today. I work alongside them, give them opportunities and responsibilities, and let them sort through problems as they encounter them.

I will offer a word of encouragement, point them in the right direction if they're clearly drifting into dangerous waters, but in the main, I trust them to do the right thing. I sincerely hope a parent who is reading this, who may have a child that has different learning needs to the majority, sees that there can be other pathways to a rewarding and hugely enjoyable life than books and academia. I do not even have a Junior or indeed Leaving Cert, God forbid college qualifications, and I have done quite alright. And so can anyone else.

The world is wide, people are generally kind and taking a chance is sometimes the best thing you can do. We can all very easily take the well-beaten path, but that rarely brings excitement and reward. Aim for the stars and you may hit the moon, but you will have fun getting there. The future is full of hope, it is positive, and it is exciting. There will be bumps, but with them comes opportunity to keep us on our toes. Everything in a life worth living is a gamble, you just need to be brave to take the first step – because that gamble might just result in one of your dreams coming true.

And that, my dear reader, is a win-win.